MMS FOR ANIMALS

MMS for Animals

A Companion Guide for the
Holistic and Autonomous Treatment
of Animals with MMS

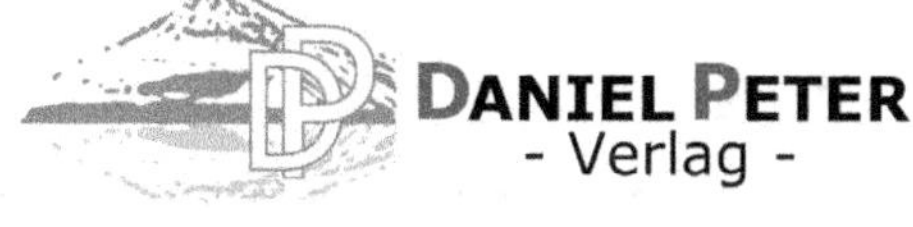

Copyright:	© 2019 by Daniel-Peter-Verlag, Schnaittach, Germany
Editing, correction and design concept:	Monika Stolina-Wolf, SONNENTOCHTER*edition*
Copy and layout:	Eva Saarbourg, Saarbourg Design
Cover design:	Markus Hoffmann, PEPP/ART. Photograph by fotolia
Thanks to:	Ulrich Bogun, Copy & Publishing Service Berlin
Translator into the English language:	Eric Gradman
Proofreading of the English language edition:	Eric Gradman
Layout of the English language edition:	Stefanie Peschetz
Publisher:	Daniel-Peter-Verlag, Schnaittach
E-Mail:	info@daniel-peter-verlag.de
Telephone orders:	+49 91 26 / 2 95 57 10
Internet:	www.daniel-peter-verlag.de
Second edition:	August 2019
ISBN	978-3-9819954-1-1

Inquiries from publishers worldwide regarding the publication of this book in the local language are most welcome!

Disclaimer

The procedures presented here are for your information only. They are not a substitute for medical diagnoses, advice, or therapies. Neither the author nor the publisher is liable for damages of any kind arising from the application of methods represented in this work. First and foremost, we accept no liability for the improvement or deterioration of the state of health of your animal.

Owing to the dynamics of the Internet the links supplied in this book that were current at the time of production of this book may have in the intervening period changed or no longer be available.

Legend: Icons

The following icons appear in this book ...

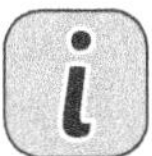 ... Information relating to topics such as medications, maladies, or research.

 ... take-home messages and particularly important information with reference to tips and tricks and relevant facts.

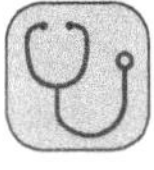 ... actual case studies from veterinary practice. The examples issue from the author Monika Rekelhof, the veterinarian Dr. Dirk Schrader, and various users whose experiences administering MMS have been chronicled in this book.

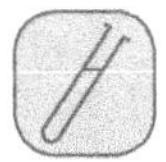 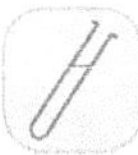 ... step by step instructions for specific dosage and provision of treatment.

Contents

1 Preface

Preface

"Animal healer with heart and soul" - precisely that was my first impression of Monika Rekelhof. Animals of all kinds and sizes, particularly their well being, are her focus, and doubtless will be so in her heart of hearts in the future. Furthermore, Monika Rekelhof is the kind of person who is not deterred by a "no way." It is this special quality that moves her to explore new avenues.

With "MMS for Animals. A Companion Guide for the Holistic and Autonomous Treatment of Animals with MMS" we have in our hands an explication of how to use MMS (Master Mineral Solution) to treat animals. Naturally, it was most gratifying to be asked by Monika to write this foreword, as, like many of my fellows, I had already for many years had good experiences myself. For all that, I too was somewhat skeptical and frightened of using MMS on our little, still young cat that at the time weighed hardly three kilogram (6.613 lb). I followed her advice in full trust, and behold: our little Marzipannäschen was already better the following day!

On every page of this book the reader can discern the author's sense of responsibility towards creatures, as well as her engagement, unperturbed by rules and limits, concerning the well being of all living entities. It is Monika Rekelhof's aspiration to achieve a complete understanding of animals whose language we scarcely comprehend and even so care for while they are under our protection. Fortuitously, by reading this book we also receive as animal owners instances of unexpected advice regarding how we might perhaps better understand ourselves, or simply treat ourselves. Into the bargain, in a friendly fashion, we gain much impetus to ponder issues such as appropriate feeding, vaccination, and natural association with animals.

"To heal beloved animals holistically and independently" - naturally the animal communication that Monika Rekelhof masterfully and assiduously deploys and passes on in courses applies. There are many things between heaven and earth that we do not understand, or do not understand right away. Yet they exist.

In the following book the author goes into the comprehensive treatment of animals with the aid of MMS, DMSO, CDS/CDS-plus in great detail, and much more.

In the first year students already learn the following in chemistry lessons: "Every chemical on earth is poisonous in large amounts."

The best example is common cooking salt, which is used by most of us daily. Think about it: A full cup is deadly! But its use is of course safe in recommended doses.

Likewise we can be certain that to drink seven Liter (1.849 gal) water in one go can kill you. The dosage is key!

Monika Rekelhof does not wish to convert anybody: Time and again she encourages reflection, questions, indicates possibilities, or reports on experiences. When you, dear readers, also like on occasion to look beyond the rim of your plate, then trust in yourself!

This book can in wonderful ways contribute and consequently hold out the possibility that our sensitivity towards our fellow creatures and ourselves is advanced in wondrous ways.

With respect to this theme, the author guides us so empathically that even the greatest skeptic can assuredly take this path concerning the good health of their animals.

Dr. h. c. Ulrike C. Hillgner
Arnheim, January 2015

2 Introduction

*I*t is my life purpose to help animals, and thus, at times, humans too. A part of this enterprise is to proceed boldly and to promote and disseminate that benedictory "agent" MMS. Even though MMS is on occasion discussed heatedly it is not my aim to prove a point, but rather, proceeding from my experiences administering MMS, and from my perspective, to clarify. Each decides for oneself and is independently responsible as to whether to make changes for oneself or their four-legged pets and actually employ a remedy such as MMS. MMS is a very effective medication in spite of all the contention. On a related note: The intent ought not be to put the veterinary profession in question. Classical Medicine and Naturopathy or Holistic Medicine have in the last ten years moved increasingly closer, and it is my express wish to work with veterinarians so that the various approaches complement one another.

Deciding to use MMS, CDS and CDSplus of their own volition autonomously

Writing this introduction brings to mind the time that the media reported at length on the so called "E Numbers" and the harmfulness of particular ingredients. These reports roused the consciousness of consumers. One would see patrons turn each product round to check the constituent ingredients. To this day these or similar E Numbers are still in use - who looks any longer? Are these substances any less hazardous today? Nowadays, who is interested when buying pre-prepared grill-meat that these E Numbers are listed there as well?

Reports about E Numbers in the media

Many things have become a matter of course and so most people proceed as though things must be just fine. There was a long struggle to develop a deposit system for glass bottles. So what do we have now? Plastic bottles! Even the media reportage concerning the environmental impact, especially in the oceans, does not help to bring change here. It was a shock for me recently when after a long time I wanted to buy lemon-

Lemonade in plastic bottles only

ade in a beverage store and could find lemonade in plastic bottles only.

It is just the same as regards animal feed. We trust the appealing and unfortunately precisely targeted advertising. But what is actually to be found inside the package? Why must flavor-enhancers, dyestuffs and sugar be added? If our animals knew what processed feed contained they would assuredly not eat it. A colleague reported that she once had a biologist privately test industrially produced feed from a leading and pricey brand for its ingredients; frighteningly, this expert confirmed the presence of sewage sludge. How would it be then if we again paid more attention to the ingredients? It is crucial in all aspects of life to formulate one's own opinions.

I would like to cite the author and journalist Hans-Ulrich Grimm who in his recent book "Katzen würden Mäuse kaufen" (Cats Would Buy Mice) heavily criticizes animal feed manufacturers. In this branch of industry there is apparently a failure of all "revulsion impediments/disgust brakes," contended Grimm on Deutschlandradio Kultur. Slaughterhouse waste and spoiled meat is repeatedly processed into meat and bone meal (MBM). Producers benefit in this way from the waste disposal problems of feed production. Large amounts of slaughterhouse waste that must somehow be disposed of are generated: "They offer this refuse to animal feed manufacturers who are grateful to receive it!" Among the scandals uncovered, manufacturers had in fact "for years processed sewage sludge into animal fodder simply because it was not prohibited."

According to Grimm the industry uses "all manner of chemical tricks" in order that the animals will accept degenerated feed. "They (the animals) are systematically led by the nose, their palate fooled with, and only by such means will they consume that stuff." The author maintains that this is not only the case with animals. In food production an "astonishing amount of taste manipulation" is undertaken, "so that the stuff that issues from factories can even be indulged."

Furthermore, the author deplores the close entanglement of scientists and the animal food industry. In the course of this research it was not possible to track down independent researchers. Most animal food studies are financed by the industry. It is, to be sure, a legitimate matter to find out what type of nutrition best suits an animal. "But only to compare assorted canned foods and to completely bypass Nature, that is surely in the interests of Industry."

Research is financed by the industry

It is as good as the same with alternative medicine. My husband and I have tried many new medications ourselves before giving them to the animals. We want to experience and thus know how the medications feel in the body, and what reactions occur in the body due to the medicines. I experiment and then decide whether it is good for me and/or the animals. There are multitudes of highly beneficial substances that are forbidden or have simply "disappeared" into the bottom draw. Now though, thank goodness, they are being rediscovered, and thanks to the Internet are again available. Some good and beneficial agents though, for example hemp, can unfortunately not be freely purchased in Germany except in special cases on prescription for pain therapy.

Test the medicine ourselves before giving it to the animals.

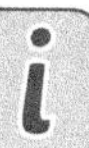

Hemp

Between 300 BC and 200 AD the first known article regarding hemp as medication is to be found in a Chinese medical text. In 1898 William Randolph Hearst by means of inflammatory tabloid reportage began his campaign to have the American government outlaw hemp. His exclusive interest was however the production of paper as back then paper was very cheaply produced from hemp and not from wood as in later times. In 1937 the use of hemp was prohibited.

It is difficult for me in this light to comprehend that it was actually possible to make hemp invisible and almost entirely disappear from public awareness in spite of the abundance of reading matter, accounts of healing, and applications. To many it is known solely as a drug.

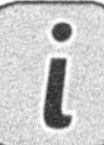

Strophanthin

Until 1960 Strophanthin was approved as a medicinal substance and rated highly as a heart medication in Germany. This pharmaceutical for the treatment of acute cardiac insufficiency was in use until 1992, yet today it has vanished from the marketplace. On what grounds?

One could list myriad substances that in times past have shown themselves to serve humanity extremely well in regard to healing and recovery. Now we come to the actual theme of this book: MMS. There are similar stories to those of strophanthin and hemp to tell that concern MMS. To follow, you will encounter more relating to this theme.

Who could profit by causing this agent to disappear little by little? How could this even happen? One thing is however certain: He that has money has the power to effect societal change.

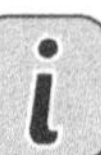

MMS

Jim Humble discovered MMS in 1996. Concomitant with being able to help thousands of people who were affected by Malaria he went public. It was also proposed that the WHO perform more extensive studies regarding the medicine; the offer though was declined. In the meantime many books and films regarding the use of MMS have appeared worldwide. Doctors, natural health practitioners, veterinarians and animal alternative health professionals employ the medication. Hundreds of thousands of reports (worldwide) giving witness that the deployment of MMS leads to full recovery can be read in books and on the Internet.

What motivated me to write this book?

A basic and principal motivation for the conception of this book is the desire, as explained above, to throw light on the ways industrially prepared feed can cause our animals to get sick and be poisoned, and, on the other hand, how with MMS there exists a wonderful opportunity to purge our animals of these poisons.

A further and even more important incentive is the helplessness of many veterinarians who often can do nothing for their fosterlings and are at wits' end in spite of their Latin. Time after time I have heard veterinarians utter sentences such as: "... your animal is beyond treatment," "... we have no recommendations," "... don't know the cause," and so on. Frequently the medications administered cause animals to be even more unwell than beforehand - while, all too often, from healing or recovery there is nothing to be heard.

The helplessness of veterinarians

And finally the unimaginable side effects of conventional medications impelled me to point out to readers alternative treatments by which our animals can be healed with no or limited side effects, or at least how significant improvement to their overall condition can be achieved. Even if the following medications and possibilities described continue to be received with disdain or opposition by the general public, it is a matter close to my heart to pass on my knowledge in accordance with my attainments, and to inform of the potentials of MMS and other natural methodologies. It would truly be a shame were this, like so much other knowledge, lost, or worse, simply kept secret. In my opinion each of us should have the right to decide independently by what means they wish to manage their own health and wellbeing along with the health and wellbeing of their animals.

Make treatment alternatives public

Among all the alternative medications I have come to know none impresses for its efficacy as does MMS. That is why it lies especially close to my heart to write of the worthwhile lessons learned, and to thereby convey this to people in order that this

Extraordinary medicinal substance discovered

medication continues to be a boon to humans and animals, especially considering that in the case of eighty percent of all animal maladies, whether attributable to bacteria, viruses or fungi, no orthodox medicines are available other than noxious antibiotics against which bacteria increasingly develop resistance even as conventional medics have not a single tenable response to viruses. "MMS for Animals" presents in a precise and detailed manner how you can safely implement this medication and thereby bring benefit to your animals.

We can steer the therapy of our animals in the right direction.

MMS is no panacea and I can no more promise (nor is it permissible to do so) a cure than can a veterinarian. It is never possible to predict how a treatment might play out; we can however orient our ministrations towards our animals in the right direction. So goes the axiom oft-quoted by veterinarians in connection with a successful operation: "Everything now lies in the hand of God!" It is good so! And being that we are all God's children we can take the project of healing into our own hands!

Monika Rekelhof
Goch, February 2015

2.1 When did this project begin?

How it all began

A question I first asked myself: When did actually I learn of MMS, Jim Humble, and all that is associated, and as a consequence make a start with my own experiments? How did I get involved initially?

A thank you to the angels

Indeed, it is no longer possible to piece this together, though as early as ten years ago I learned "by chance" of Jim Humble and his discovery of MMS. Probably, it was while conversing with an acquaintance at a bathing lake in Bavaria. Was it really by chance? If so, then I am still gratified and thankful. Needless to say, a big thank you to the angels that orchestrated all this!

What I heard would not leave me be. So I sat myself down at home at the computer and investigated by way of Google. What I read there intrigued me all the more: I wanted to experience more concerning this substance. I immediately purchased Jim Humble's book "MMS - Breakthrough," and shortly after performed the first experiments on myself.

The genesis: "MMS - Breakthrough" by Jim Humble

Seeing that increasing to fifteen drops is mentioned in the first book, I too naturally wanted to arrive at that number - I am unfortunately over zealous in such matters and ignore the guidelines. I must confess it was ghastly. The flavor of the mixture seemed to me like I had drunken water from the swimming pool, or worse. I could not get rid of the smell of chlorine. I had the feeling it was everywhere in my nose. As I also paid no heed to the initial reactions such as a rumbling stomach and a light queasiness, and eagerly bumped up the dose (in larger steps than advised), this was then the outcome: I spent a whole day on the toilet. Just as with medicine, one ought comply with the instructions. Medicine as well can trigger strong reactions when one does not take note of the advice in the patient information leaflet. Nonetheless, it was a beneficial experience. The effects of my actions were surprising: Already the next day I felt splendid, and being that it was my own mistake the fallout did not discourage me - quite the opposite. I use MMS to this day with a little more caution and smaller doses of course, and thanks to CDS and CDSplus, a gentler upgrade of MMS incorporating the same active agent, it is very easy to handle (without a day on the toilet!). With CDS and CDSplus the taste and reactions to the active ingredient such as diarrhea and regurgitation can be avoided. (By the by: To all those that cry, "There! See! You get diarrhea!" I would like to make plain that I react in the same way to antibiotics and other medicines, if not worse!) Afterwards, I had myself examined by my family doctor who confirmed that I have not been so healthy in a long while.

Initial experiments on myself

Too much ambition brings no good…

CDSplus, the milder alternative

Whether allergy, cold, thrush, mosquito bite, herpes: everything goes away with MMS.

As one might expect the subsequent tests were for me even greater successes. Allergies, cold, vaginal mycosis, mosquito bites, herpes: all vanish with MMS. This medication was for me simply awe-inspiring, and I am most thankful to have been granted the courage to try it out. Best of all, my husband and I no longer fear being ill or our animals getting sick.

No more fear of sickness

Somewhat later, due to necessity, one of our cats was allowed to test MMS. I was astonished to see our Sunshine lick the MMS thinned with water from the floor. Since then this medicine has become a permanent feature when treating animals. We have two dogs, two cats and two alpacas: all have been administered MMS at one time or another, and are healthy and lively.

The courage to be autonomous

Of course, the decision to choose this form of treatment is not always easy to make on one's own. One must and is entitled to decide for oneself, no one should deny this somebody. Since we from childhood on have mostly never learnt to make decisions regarding our own health or that of our animals, but are instead conditioned to surrender the responsibility for our health to doctors, a degree of courage together with some study is required before taking up the rudder for oneself. Just as MMS is not a stand-alone "miracle cure," this does not however mean dispensing with a visit to the veterinarian! That said, it is important to know that MMS is a "killer" for bacteria, viruses and parasites, and in this capacity, in the view of animal owners, it works wonders many a time.

Implementation of MMS, CDS, CDSplus, and DMSO has become routine at my practice for animal medicine.

The implementation of MMS, CDS and CDSplus has become routine with regard to my practice of animal medicine, assisting me in healing animals. This, though, is only when the owners are expressly decided and give approval. They are thereby enabled to share responsibility for the treatment of their animal in my practice.

It would give me pleasure by means of this book to demonstrate what a "water conditioner" (the original application for MMS is to condition water) can accomplish and embolden you to utilize alternative approaches to animal medicine. It is important to me that therapies and diagnoses not be accepted as self-evident but be questioned when it is called for. It makes no sense to me to cause animals to become longtime dependent, or to engender chronic disorders owing to the medication. Certainly, many of the therapeutic approaches employed by classical medicine make sense and are justifiable. But who asks what the constituents of the injection that the animal receives at the veterinarian are, what the specific ingredients are, and whether there might be side effects? Most animal owners shrug their shoulders when I ask what the veterinarian injected their animal with. The reason for the visit to the veterinarian is a particular problem, but before a diagnosis is even made an injection is administered. Generally this is a broad-spectrum antibiotic, and in some cases a painkiller. Initially the medication may in fact be effective in that the symptoms are mitigated. Is the animal healed though? Does it get to the root causes? I would like here to proffer an example as to what causal investigation (etiology) entails in my view, and how in many instances one can better help without medication:

Ask about the side effects of the medication!

Combating the symptoms or investigating the causes?

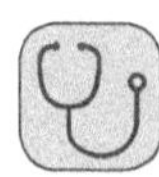

A medium-size dog exhibiting signs of paralysis of the hind legs

A medium-sized dog of approximately six years of age exhibited signs of paralysis in the hind legs. Lengthy walks were as a rule not possible. Diagnosis by the veterinarian: Incipient osteoarthritis (arthrosis). The dog was given medication, and when it was really bad, injected with a painkiller. Being that the dog-owners were not prepared to continue this treatment indefinitely, they came to me one day. I listened carefully, and posed questions: recent vaccinations and feeding habits being among them. On this basis I recommended that the owners change the dog's diet to BARF (biologically species-appropriate raw meat feeding). In addition the dog underwent an energy treatment to release blockages and restore the flow of energies. When I informed them that the dog needed nothing further presently they shook their heads in disbelief. About three weeks later the owners admitted that they had only gone partway with the new diet as they still had an almost full sack of "good, expensive dehydrated food." Astoundingly, at this point in time the

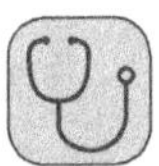

> **Continuation: A medium-size dog exhibiting signs of paralysis of the hind legs**
>
> dog was already doing much better! Subsequent to a period of complete change of diet the symptoms totally vanished. To my great delight I sometimes see the dog on walks. This example should in no way persuade you to never visit a veterinarian. Have the vet or therapist clarify the diagnosis, and then decide for yourself how the treatment should proceed!

2.2 How did I finally come to write this book?

I had a dream …

It all began with a dream. One night I dreamed of Jim Humble. He requested I write a book for him. I replied: "That's ridiculous! A book about animals exists already. Why then should I write one?" The beauty of such dreams is that you can converse in Bavarian with no problems of understanding! It was instantly clear to me that we were talking about a book for animals. Jim Humble was resolute. He repeated loud and clear: "Write me a book!" When I woke in the morning I thought: "So ein Schmarrn!" (Bavarian for: "What nonsense!"). "Me! Write a book! And such an important subject!"

Many a time things come to pass otherwise as one might imagine …

The unexpected request from the Daniel-Peter-Verlag only a few days after my dream

By dint of my work with MMS in my medical practice for animals, and due to the book "The MMS Handbook" by Dr. Antje Oswald I came into contact with the Daniel-Peter-Verlag. In November 2013 I received an unexpected email from Daniel Peter, or rather from his co-worker Gabriela that would change my life. Daniel Peter asked whether I would write a book about MMS and its use with animals. Yes, and what shall I tell you? This came about only days after my dream!

My initial reaction was: "Oh God! Me? Oh no! Am I able to do such a thing anyway?" This and other questions whizzed round my head. Following the first, lengthy, and very pleasant conversation with Daniel Peter the two of us agreed that I should simply begin writing and then we would see. After all, I had already amassed considerable practical knowledge in respect to MMS. The first spontaneous pages were written and sent to Daniel Peter to read - he liked what he saw.

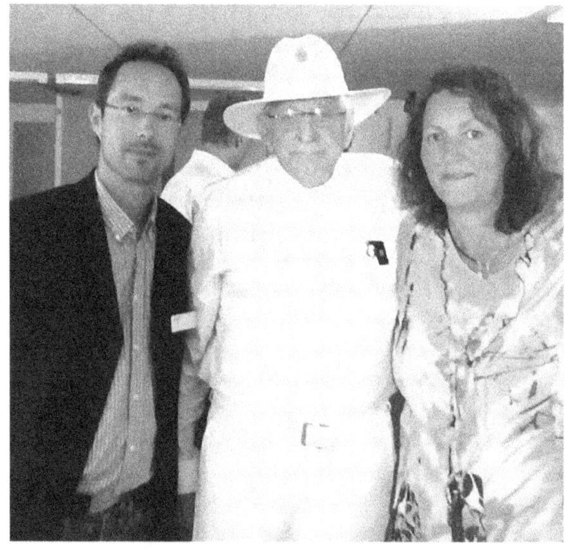

Daniel Peter, Jim Humble, Monika Rekelhof

So we took the next step and signed the writer's contract at the "Spirit of Health" Congress 2014 in Hannover. The go-ahead for the book was now official; a new and tremendously exciting step for me. Since that day in April I have come to know ever more new people who work with MMS and provide keen support for the book by passing on their experiences. Now dear readers you hold this book in your hands; so begins another exciting episode!

Signing of the writer's contract at the "Spirit of Health" Congress 2014

Something more I would like to point out is that "MMS for Animals. A Companion Guide for the Holistic and Autonomous Treatment of Animals with MMS" is not intended to be a scientific or medical textbook. The book conveys in plain language how to go about using MMS, clarifying the first steps towards its administration on one's own authority. Should you be uncertain or have questions please make contact with a therapist or veterinarian who has experience with this medicine, or is at least open-minded. You will find several therapists and veterinarians listed at end of the book.

May the book you have in your hands make your first steps easy.

I wish to offer my special thanks to Jim Humble, Dr. Andreas Kalcker, Leo Koehof and Dr. Hartmut Fischer, and the countless comrades-in-arms for their tireless commitment,

Thanks to Jim Humble, Dr. Andreas Kalcker, Leo Koehof and Dr. Hartmut Fischer

propelling the research forward. Due to the engagement of many people MMS, CDS, CDSplus and DMSO could be made accessible to the general public, and be distributed worldwide. It was especially gratifying to personally meet Jim Humble, Dr. Andreas Kalcker and Dr. Hartmut Fischer in Hannover, April 2014.

3 Holistic Medicine

For me "Alternative Medicine" is not just an alternative to medicine, but an all-embracing perspective regarding the living being animal. What is the background to holistic medicine? What do I understand holistic medicine to be?

Alternative medicine - the holistic perspective as regards the individual living being

It is very important to perceive each animal as a unique individual. Every animal is something very special in itself. Hence various methods of healing are applicable when approaching treatment, yet in many cases there are subtle differences that may prolong or even obstruct the process of healing. These manifest according to the specific case. Each therapy has its own effect on a particular animal! The standard protocols and case studies in this book are examples of potential treatments. There are cases where minimal, yet subtle differences can prolong or even preclude the healing process; in such instances please consult a veterinarian or therapist who can negotiate the subtleties.

Each animal must be viewed as a unique individual.

By means of a systematic anamnesis (a complete recalling to memory) I attempt to trace the cause of the illness. At first questions concerning nutrition, vaccinations and deworming are posed to uncover how the ailments may have arisen. Furthermore, it is important to find out about an animal's origins. Did it come from an animal shelter or from abroad? Has it previously had many owners? Has there been serious change or great misfortune in its environs? Has the animal any afflictions stemming from operations or diseases? Is the animal on medication? This is where it begins, and then proceeds to more specific matters.

The treatment begins with anamnesis.

Generally, the first consideration with anamnesis is nutrition. Nutrition is crucial, because daily nutrition can cause many problems and even diseases. Animals receive lots of poor quality proteins with industrially produced feed.

Substandard protein in industrial feed

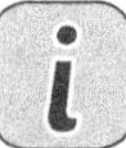

What does the intake of low grade protein engender?

Heating to above 40°C (104°F) tear apart the amino acid chains that are component parts of proteins, thus destroying the whole structure of the protein - the higher the temperature, the more the damage. The consequence is over acidification of the blood leading to a subsequent reduction in oxygen transport, and thus undernourishment of the organs. This undernourishment of the tissue usually results in the medical condition osteoarthritis. In most cases osteoarthritis is not a consequence of overload due to movement but the outcome of a poorly functioning metabolism due to deficient nutrition.

Animals receive loads of substandard protein in industrially prepared feed.

Milieu and sanitation

Another issue that I think is important presently is the milieu (of the metabolism), and the sanitation thereof. Please note: Milieu does not in this case represent filth, dirt or slums. Heating meat damages important nutrients. Due to the structural modifications of the proteins in the degraded metabolic processes, ammonia in the liver and nitrogen in the kidneys are increasingly released and exuded as urea via the kidneys. Many ailments originate in the metabolism and subsequently lead to kidney dysfunction; I often must deal with the repercussions in my practice, mostly with cats. Muscle disorders ensue with this increased elimination of ammonia. The heart too being a muscle the implications are not difficult to envision.

What more can disturb the balance of the inner milieu? To follow are a few important examples:

Heavy metals in vaccines and drinking vessels

Included are stresses attributable to heavy metals such as quicksilver, aluminum, cadmium, lead, copper and nickel. Some, for example, quicksilver and aluminum are commonly to be found in large amounts in vaccines. Often animals' drinking and feeding dishes are made from aluminum. Since small amounts of aluminum are being released continually it is preferable to change over to ceramic or porcelain dishes.

Toxins caused by bacteria and parasites - endotoxins - may be present. Endotoxins are formed through the disruption of specific bacteria (coliform bacteria, salmonella et cetera). For example, fever may occur as a consequence. Issues relating to endotoxins are common in the stalls of high-performance cows. Symptoms may be infections of the udder, metritis, and hoof and claw diseases. For horse owners and milk-cow farmers it is important to know that problems relating to botolinum toxins may be brought about by feeding with baled silage. These toxins develop when the cadaver of a mouse is wrapped into the bale. Botolinum toxins count among the most dangerous poisons known to nature.

Difficulties caused by endotoxins

Another important consideration is man-made environmental toxins such as wood preservatives, insecticides, dioxins, and plastics. Even small amounts, for example, the remains of a mouse that has eaten in a field sprayed with pesticides, can poison a cat that has eaten this mouse. Neither should you allow your dog to run out onto sprayed fields as the paws may pick up insecticides; when it licks its paws these toxic substances enter directly into the bloodstream. You will certainly recall the scandals over animal fodder contaminated by dioxins, as well as that concerning dioxinated eggs. Even if they are no longer written or talked about this does not mean that the dangers no longer exist. Quite the opposite: These environmental toxins can be extremely harmful to our animals.

Environmental pollutants in the food chain

Further substances harmful to the body are preservatives and flavor enhancers. Producers endeavor to prolong the storage periods for foods, but the same problem arises as regards industrially produced animal fodder as with some pre-prepared meals for humans: this is not wholesome, engendering ill health.

Preservatives and flavor enhancers

Hormones, anti-biotics, chlorine and toxic metals

Hormones, antibiotics, chlorine and toxic metals in drinking water are similarly problematic.

Radiation

Many animals exhibit disorders and physical damage due to exposure to electrosmog.

Exhaust fumes

Another important consideration with regard to anamnesis is environmental pollution. Among these pollutants are exhaust gases from cars and factories, pesticides, and residues of pharmaceuticals in drinking water. Residues from the following pharmaceuticals have been detected in high quantities: The diabetes medication Metformin and the antibiotic Tamiflu for treating colds and flu. These medications are not broken down by the organism and are disposed of in the urine. Not to be overlooked are substances such as plastics and residues of hormones (the "Pill") in the water. These stress the metabolism, ergo the organs of humans and animals.

Hormone residues in the water

Therefore, provide your animals with filtered water. It is possible that there is a chemical plant nearby to your dwelling and that the contaminants propagate serious organic disorders. Maybe you live in a city and walk your dog through the streets where your dog gets the full load of exhaust emissions. The animals take in these and other pollutants from sources including air and water, even grass.

> MMS can help rein in the effects of these poisons to an extraordinary degree. It oxidizes pathogens and heavy metals and also has a positive effect on the milieu. As pathogenic agents reside mainly in an acidic "subverted" milieu, on account of nutritional deficiencies for instance, an antioxidant such as MMS can adjust the pH value and thus improve the milieu by supplying the tissue with oxygen.

Dietary change

Changes to nutrition must be undertaken at one and the same time. You will find further information on the subject of nutrition in Chapter 9.

To ascertain the points at issue for each particular animal an extended anamnesis is crucial. This entails allowing enough time and calm for a detailed recalling to memory with the owners. Naturally, dialogue with the animal itself is essential. This frequently gets to the point!

Additional sources of animal infirmities, though often still considered to be laughable, are the effects of electrosmog, disturbance caused by water veins, and other stresses hidden to the eye.

Electrosmog, disturbance due to water veins

Animals either avoid radiation or they seek it out. More about this in Chapter 14 "Animal Communication." Cows and horses avoid radiation. In former times, for this reason, informed by the powerful instincts of animals, farmers would build stables and housing on sites where radiation was low. They observed their herds in the fields and watched where the animals would gather and settle to sleep. They built in these locations. These days we often force our animals to rest in places that are not beneficial to them only because this might be visually the "nicest" spot for the doggy basket or the like. The continual stress brought on by various emissions or electrosmog can modify the blood for instance. Excessive cellphone usage is known to cause Rouleaux formation in the blood of humans.

Animals: Avoiders or seekers of radiation

Rouleaux formation in the blood caused by radiation

What is a Roulex formation?

Everyone has of course heard of red blood cells, the Erythrocytes. The typical red color of blood obtains from these. Through a microscope round discs of identical size, indented at the center, are to be seen.

When exposed to electromagnetic waves the erythrocytes adhere to one another in a formation called Rouleaux. The surface area is diminished considerably on account of this grouping; absorption of oxygen is thus restricted. The large chains of these grouped erythrocytes cannot pass through the fine veins causing hypoxemia. The cells in consequence acidify as is reflected by the pH value.

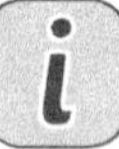

It is not possible within the frame of a book like "MMS for Animals" to specify and adequately investigate every pertinent environmental contaminant such as plastic. An objective of this book is to provide stimulus to search out information, to consult the Web, and to dissuade you from being misguided and confused by the pretty advertisements or beguiling slogans. These have but one purpose: To swill megabucks into the coffers of pharmaceutical and food industries. Their revenues are enormous as evidenced by the following two examples. These and other sales figures data can be found in the Internet. Be inquisitive and take a look at the sites of some familiar firms.

Profit maximization rather than maintenance of health

Pfizer Inc., that, among other products, produces an antibiotic (Synolux RTU) for animals, has an annual turnover internationally of US$ 51.6 billion!

Mars Inc., manufacturer of the popular brands Cesar, Chappi, Dreamies, Frolic, Greenies, James Wellbeloved, Kitekat, Loyal, Nutro, Pedigree, Perfect Fit, Royal Canin, Sheba, Trill, Whiskas, and Winergy, realized an annual turnover in the order of US$ 33 billion in 2011.

Of course one cannot take as read bad intentions on the basis of the sales figures of these corporations. The mindful reader will be aware though that the primary concern for the managers of these firms is not healthy nutrition for animals, or their general wellbeing, but simply the maximization of profits. It is important to be awake to this when choosing food products or medication for your animal.

Psychological stress for animals

We now arrive at an all-important dimension as regards the anamnesis of your animals. In the framework of holistic medicine all issues concerning the emotions and the psyche are of great consequence. Here it is essential to employ animal communication in order to gain information regarding the animal and its psychological makeup. More on the theme of "Animal Communication" can be found in Chapter 14. The same signs manifest frequently: People subject to occupational stress exhibit gastrointestinal problems, as do animals that suffer diarrhea or the like.

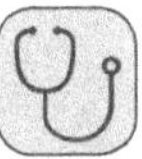

A female dog with recurring inflammation of the urinary bladder

The first case concerns a bitch suffering persistently recurring cystitis. Each time the dog suffered this symptom the owner exhibited signs of nervous stress that she sought to dull with alcohol. In this situation only a focused energetic buffer from the owner could bring relief. Acute irritations could be healed with MMS, colloidal silver, and homeopathic medicine.

Unstable people usually have unstable animals. This creates permanent stress, and over the years the pendulum swings higher and higher - this can be detrimental to the metabolism. Due to this contiguity animals react with rashes or gastrointestinal ailments.

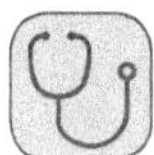

A female cat with behavioral problems

The second example relates to a cat that according to her owner repeatedly urinates in the strangest of places. The veterinarian was unable to establish a cause. All tests were favorable - the cat was healthy. In the course of an exhaustive interview the owner told me that her husband was often away at work for long periods. She mentioned that the cat had a number of times peed in his suitcase. By means of animal communication the cat told me I ought ask the woman how it was for her when her husband was absent. I myself supposed that the woman felt poorly under these circumstances, but on my asking she gave a disturbing response: She was relieved each time he went for he was an alcoholic and as a result often became aggressive. It turned out that the situation with her son was similar. Sadly, she would not or could not instigate change in the short term. She later told me that she visited another veterinarian who administered hormonal treatment that for a short time reduced the urination activities of the cat. The problem did not end with that: To compensate for the hormonal treatment the cat's brother sprang to the fore and peed in various spots in her place! Meeting the woman one time by chance I asked whether her situation had in someway changed. She told me that she had purchased a new kitchen. There is nothing more to be said ...

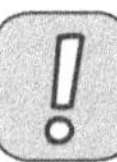

To detect the source of an illness, it is imperative to consider the animal's environment in totality.

The categories "Diet," "Vaccination," and "The Animal's Environment" aid me greatly in pushing forward with each anamnesis. In depth information regarding these themes is to be found in the chapters to come.

Being that in many cases the correspondence between human and animal is self-evident, the correlation of equivalent clinical delineations is assumed. Accordingly, animal owners often ask me whether they ought take MMS themselves: It may well be a good idea, but then the decision must be their own.

One thing is always especially important, I believe: No animal is the same as another. I view each animal as a one of a kind living organism and render the respect due by taking the time to consider its individual concerns for it is inherently the interaction of body, mind, and soul that keeps our animals healthy.

3.1 The work at my medical practice for animals

The holistic treatment of animals

Obviously, in my practice I treat the animals holistically. By means of animal communication I look to identify the source of as well as the trigger for the malady. Alongside therapies involving homeopathy, Schüssler Salts, plant-based tinctures, and needless to say MMS, CDS and CDSplus it is critical that a species-appropriate diet be incorporated.

"Can I give that to my animal?" This is one of the most common questions at my practice.

I am frequently greeted with skepticism when I recommend MMS, CDS or CDSplus. Clients pose questions such as: Can I give it to my animal? It reeks of chlorine, isn't it poisonous? What! I should give my animal an antiseptic for water? I read some negative stuff in the news and in the Internet, and I ought administer that? I cheerfully put a few drops of CDS on the back of my hand, rub it in, and thus demonstrate that the substance is not, as the media claims, "corrosive." (One can do this with only CDS of course, and not with undiluted MMS!) Then, to allay anxieties and prejudices, I speak extensively with my clients, citing the best-known books on the subject. Often the biggest fears concern the taking of new paths, shaking off conformity in order to arrive at decisions other than the familiar and habitual. Of course the clients themselves come to the decision

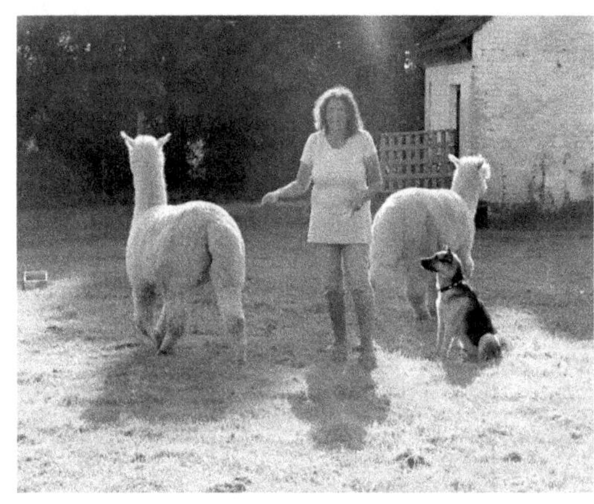

Spirit, Duncan, Paco, and Monika Rekelhof in the middle

of whether or not to dispense this medicine. I advise all my clients that as a basic principle it is their own responsibility when making such a decision, with maximum backup naturally. I often encourage clients to pragmatically weigh up the side effects and indications provided on the classic patient information leaflet relative to the known adverse reactions to for instance MMS (as described earlier).

Qualms and anxieties brought into positive alignment by means of information and intuition…

Chlorine dioxide is formed from sodium chlorite; therefore a main constituent of MMS/CDS and CDSplus, as we now learned, is sodium chlorite. When one searches the Internet for "sodium chlorite," of course one often lands on MMS and CDS. In addition, the astonishing medical bulletins from Afghanistan by the medical practitioner Prof. Dr. Kurt-W. Stahl are disseminated there. The professor employs Sodium chlorosum to treat his patients who are infected with cutaneous leishmaniasis. Sodium chlorosum is the pharmaceutical name for sodium chlorite.

Chlorine dioxide is formed from sodium chlorite.

4 MMS - The Theoretical Part

4.1 What is MMS?

What actually is MMS and what does it do in our animal's body? "MMS" is the acronym for "Master Mineral Solution." Chlorine dioxide is an active agent that is usually made up of two components.

"MMS" is the acronym for "Master Mineral Solution".

One component is the base substance Sodium chlorite solution and the other an acid. This sodium chlorite (NaClO2) should not be mistaken for common cooking salt (NaCl = Sodium chloride). When sodium chlorite (NaClO2) is mixed with an acid it releases the actual active agent Chlorine dioxide.

A sodium chlorite solution and an acid constitute the base components of MMS

Chlorine dioxide (CLO2) is an oxidant. Oxidation is a natural process whereby the human body, in the lungs for example, eradicates pathogens with oxygen; electrons are extracted from the pathogens causing them to simply break apart. This is also the reason bacteria cannot develop resistance to chlorine dioxide. With orthodox medicine antibiotics are used to combat bacteria. Antibiotics are poisonous substances that are anabolicly absorbed by bacteria, that are taken in via the metabolism. There is sufficient time during this process for information to be transferred to the genetic material thus bringing about resistances. Chlorine dioxide, conversely, eradicates pathogenic agents through oxidation; the bacteria are defenseless. Chlorine dioxide even eliminates pathogenic viruses in this way, which is remarkable considering that orthodox western medicine knows of not a single medication to counter viruses.

Chlorine dioxide (ClO2) is an oxidant.

Bacteria and viruses cannot develop resistance to MMS.

MMS eliminates even viruses.

Bacteria and viruses cannot develop resistance to MMS (chlorine dioxide)!

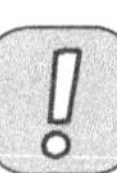

4.1.1 How do I envisage the effect of MMS?

MMS can transport oxygen to body liquids.

A pond that is not supplied enough oxygen develops into a fermenting, stinking slough full of pathogens. Pathogenic agents can similarly attack the human body, which is composed of more than 70% water, when the water fouls. Consequently, with MMS, which is a substance that supplies oxygen to the water in the body and by means of oxidation kills germs in water, I can "oxidize" germs just as in a glass of water. Another positive effect of MMS is that it can stimulate the appetite of sick animals, hence their digestion. As MMS can eliminate pathogens in the body, the immune system is reinforced releasing considerable energy, which is then available for the task of counteracting potential disorders and assisting the processes of healing.

MMS can stimulate animals' appetite and support their immune system.

For a better understanding you also can read the reports deriving from my animal practice in Chapter 7, as well as reports by other therapists and private individuals. I am especially grateful to these dedicated people. They have selflessly contributed to this work and enabled me to learn many new things. It is heartening to repeatedly be given the opportunity to get to know such interesting and courageous people owing to this work, plus those I will no doubt meet further along the way. By this means I continue to receive fresh impulses to proceed with and advance my work. A healthy animal is always the greatest reward for doing this work.

The greatest reward is a healthy animal.

Against which disorders is MMS helpful?

I have been asked many times by animal owners when it might be appropriate to contact me regards sick animals. You may have similar queries concerning MMS and CDS. Which symptoms or maladies occasion the administering of MMS to my animal? What can it bring? The ailments are typically virally or bacterially induced.

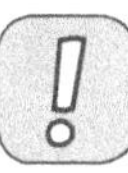

Orthodox medicine does not have a single medication to combat viral diseases; antibiotics are only effective, if at all, against bacterial diseases. Chlorine dioxide (MMS, CDS, CDSplus) eradicates viruses without any problems.

Antibiotics only help, if at all, against bacteria. Often poisoning cannot be detected right away, in the case of an attack where epilepsy is suspected for example. There are no tests for epilepsy. The cause of the attack can only be ascertained through a process of elimination. The procedure is elaborate and thus costly. Such attacks are caused by poisoning or vaccinations in many cases, and can therefore be readily treated. The same goes for some kinds of ataxia. Treatment varies from animal to animal in both instances; the therapy must be approached holistically.

Poisoning or vaccinations often bring on attacks of epilepsy.

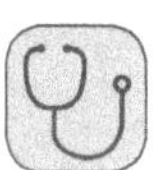

A cat diagnosed with epilepsy

A cat diagnosed with epilepsy was brought to my practice. She was treated by her veterinarian with psychotropic drugs. When I looked at her in her own home I saw a very insecure cat. Once, when looking to jump up onto a small closet, she missed her aim. By means of animal communication she signaled the root of her disorder. She had eaten a moth that had come in via the window.

It was a clear-cut case of poisoning to me. She was beside herself, in the true sense of the term, due to the medication. She also relayed this to me via animal communication. Following the diagnosis the owner and I agreed upon the treatment to follow. The medication would be slowly reduced; simultaneously MMS would be employed to neutralize the poisoning and eliminate contaminants including those from the medications. Two days later the owner told me by phone that she had stopped administering the psychotropics on short notice. It was gratifying that the ongoing treatment resulted in a speedy recovery. The cat suffered no further attacks even though the medications were discontinued.

Viral diseases such as leishmaniasis or Lyme borreliosis can be treated very effectively with MMS.

Many diseases can be treated effectively with MMS. Often it is viral diseases such as leishmaniasis. Lyme disease, a viral infection that often occurs with dogs, can be treated successfully with MMS as well. Cats frequently suffer from kidney disorders; breathing issues and mites often transpire with horses. As with humans allergies, which may be attended by dermatophytosis have become prevalent with animals. MMS can be used to treat these skin disorders with favorable outcomes.

Specific diseases and differentiated methods of treatment can be found in Chapter 7.

To enumerate the full extent of possible treatments would certainly burst the boundaries of this book, and make for reader fatigue. Individual diseases will be detailed in the animal-specific sections, though even there it is not possible to reference everything. This book compromises the largest practicable range of methods for treatment.

Just as with animals MMS can be dispensed to humans

Many questions have undoubtedly been left open thus far. In the following I would like to clarify as many of these as possible and thus simplify your approach to this curative. I am frequently made aware that animal owners already know about MMS. They have even used it themselves for a while without encountering problems, yet as soon as their own animal gets sick they contact me in distress to ask whether MMS would also be good in that particular situation!

In the book "CDS/MMS Health is Possible" (CDS/MMS Heilung ist möglich) by Dr. Andreas Kalcker I read with amazement that he initially administered MMS to his dog, and only when he saw the old fella jumping about in a manner it had not done for a long while did he dare take it himself. With me it is the reverse: I first administer a substance to my animals after I know how the human body responds.

On the basis of the examples in Chapter 7 you can see how MMS, CDS and CDSplus can be applied. It will soon become evident that these are not the only remedies available. Often the dosage varies significantly as well. I have added a few symptoms that illustrate the origins of the ailment and the ensuing developments as clarification. The practical examples represent only a sample of the manifold examples available. In addition, there are many more potential applications. In the event of your darling being unwell please consult a veterinarian or therapist first, and then agree on methods of treatment and dosage. If a condition goes unmentioned in this book, this does not mean MMS might not work.

After reviewing the medical history, and perhaps talking with the animal, all factors are aggregated. It can now be decided how the therapy should proceed. Potential medication is tested and the dosage determined. When the owners have acquired all the medications for the animal treatment can begin. It is crucial to me that following the first treatment I be accessible in order to provide the owners with advice and assistance, particularly in situations where anxieties, questions, or complications exist.

After reviewing the medical history the plan for treatment can be set out.

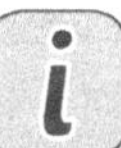

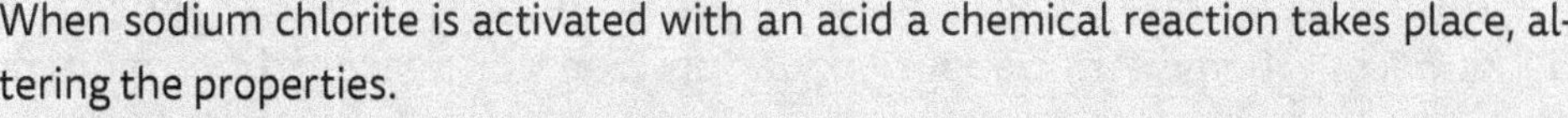

When sodium chlorite is activated with an acid a chemical reaction takes place, altering the properties.
Chlorine dioxide is a dependable killer of bacteria. Drinking the mixture causes the chlorine dioxide to enter the gastrointestinal tract and then the circulatory system. The red blood cells interpret it to be an oxygen molecule and carry it. This of course aids transport of the oxidizer to the site of the dysfunction, a great advantage relative to other substances that are not transportable by red blood cells. When the chlorine dioxide molecule meets a pathogenic agent that is sensitive to oxidation it extracts electrons from the pathogen causing it to disintegrate and be disposed of by the body as waste. By this process MMS functions as an antibacterial, antifungal, antiviral, and anti-inflammatory agent, balancing pH levels as well.

4.1.2 What is the difference between chlorine and chlorine dioxide?

Chlorine dioxide has NOTHING in common with everyday chlorine cleansers!

Chlorine dioxide does indeed smell like chlorine, yet it has nothing in common with everyday chlorine detergents with which the media likes to confuse it (MMS) thus stirring panic. Chlorine destroys pathogens by combining substances that form new substances that cause cancer. Chlorine dioxide, by contrast, destroys pathogens through the natural process of oxidation explained above.

Iodine, hydrogen peroxide, oxygen, and ozone are oxidizing agents that have long been used in medicine.

An oxidant has the potential to release oxygen and electrons, and, for instance, to absorb pathogens. At this point I would like to list some examples of substances that oxidize which are already applied in medicine and alternative medicine: iodine, hydrogen peroxide, oxygen, and ozone.

Ozone, a powerful oxidant, is nevertheless not harmful.

Ozone is a considerably stronger than chlorine dioxide. If you pour a tiny drop onto a rubber glove a hole will appear immediately. Yet doctors and alternative practitioners infuse ozone into the blood without causing damage. How can that be? The body can manage oxidation. For this reason these oxidizing substances are permitted in our drinking water and are classified as not harmful to humans and animals when diluted.

Chlorine dioxide (ClO2) has nothing in common with chlorine (Cl). Chlorine destroys pathogens by combining substances to form new substances that cause cancer. Chlorine dioxide, by contrast, destroys pathogens through oxidation, a natural process for living organisms.

Substances such as arsenic are employed in alternative medicine as well.

Some say that chlorine dioxide is not a naturopathic remedy. Yet even in naturopathy there are substances such as arsenic, which is a chemical element and is often employed in homeopathy. Further information can be found in the book: "The MMS Handbook" by Dr. Antje Oswald (See: Bibliography).

Chlorine dioxide, the active agent in MMS, CDS and CDSplus, is only permitted as a disinfectant for water in Germany. As to the pros and cons concerning the ingestion of MMS, CDS or CDSplus it is for each of us to decide. There are medical patents relating to this topic, some of which can read at the end of this book (See: Bibliography).

So here we are dealing with a chlorine dioxide solution that has nothing in common with chlorine. Chlorine is a single element, whereas chlorine dioxide is a compound; though chemically related they differ inherently. The difference is as pronounced as for instance the difference between hydrogen and the compound of hydrogen, which we all know as water. Chlorine dioxide has completely different characteristics to chlorine. Chlorine dioxide is an oxidant that our body and that of our animals can handle very well. Blood transports oxygen and therefore, unlike bacteria, we are well protected against oxidation. As opposed to antibiotics, bacteria cannot form resistances to chlorine dioxide. This is of the utmost importance nowadays, as there are reports of new bacteria that have grown immune to antibiotics almost daily. These are just a few aspects. The effects and the precise correlations are graphically presented in the film "Understanding MMS" that can be purchased from publishers Daniel-Peter-Verlag.

Chlorine dioxide has totally different characteristics to chlorine.

Documentary film: "Understanding MMS"

Sodium chlorite activated with an acid is caustic and would do harm if ingested undiluted.
In the media it is repeatedly stated that the substance produced when MMS and an acid are mixed is injurious. That it is not the activated MMS that is to be digested, but a solution considerably thinned down with water is principally overlooked! I refer you to the LD50 data in Chapter 4.2.2.

Activated MMS is not drinkable, only the solution diluted in water!

Obviously, being an oxidant, chlorine dioxide is bleaching when **undiluted.** This is characteristic of oxidants. When fabric is exposed to sun and air long enough the colors bleach. Therefore

Only undiluted chlorine dioxide acts as bleach.

one should take care when handling undiluted MMS that none comes in contact with clothing. Of course you can use this attribute to remove stains from white fabric. You need only to activate undiluted MMS in a spray bottle and spray it onto the stains. This preparation is ideal for removing mildew from walls.

MMS is, for example, activated with citric acid (or hydrochloric acid, or tartaric acid), or use the ready-made mixture CDS - all in combination with water.

> **Never drink MMS pure. It is caustic in this state!**

4.1.3 Applications for chlorine dioxide

When chlorine dioxide is applied it is not possible for resistant bacteria to develop.

Chlorine dioxide destroys viruses, bacteria and fungi while producing atomic oxygen (O1), the poliovirus already at a concentration of less than 1 ppm for example. By destroying the guanine nucleotide alkalines of the liberated RNS and DNS the formation of new generations of pathogens is reliably arrested. Thus resistant strains cannot be formed. With antibiotics this transpires daily (e.g., antibiotic resistant pathogens in hospitals) rendering doctors clueless. Yet chlorine dioxide is non-cell toxic! As indications, various viral and bacterial infections as well as mycosis are referenced, and the consequences of therapies with antibiotics. No counter indications are known.[1]

There are many further studies and treatises regarding chlorine dioxide in which the extraordinary effects and successes, combating bacteria for instance, are illustrated.

Chlorine dioxide is used for disinfection in hospitals. Even in sewage purification plants it is used to eradicate bacteria from

---

1   www.seegartenklinik.ch/search=dixychlor, 15.01.2015.

drinking water. Fruit, vegetables, and meat are commonly treated with chlorine dioxide to kill pathogens and bacteria thereby extending shelf life; most everybody takes in chlorine dioxide daily. Regrettably, chlorine dioxide is relatively expensive, which is why many communities choose to employ the dangerous chlorine to purify their drinking water. The Medical Tribune in an article of 2011 states: "According to the manufacturer's data the new substance functions independently of temperature. High temperatures are no longer necessary to reduce pathogens. Thus the substance is compliant to the requirements of categories A to D of the Robert Koch Institute".[1] In reality, the "new substance" has been known for decades.

Chlorine dioxide is used in purification plants to rid the drinking water of bacteria.

Chlorine dioxide is permissible for human use including in the preparation of foodstuffs, yet if I use the term MMS for the self-same chemical public authorities and the media scream out loud that this substance is dangerous and poisonous. When I use the identical agent (chlorine dioxide) to disinfect drinking water that is approved. Is nomenclature the problem? Should we in the future only speak of chlorine dioxide (or CDS = chlorine dioxide solution)? MMS is simply the name thought up by Jim Humble. The medical application of chlorine dioxide is much older. Jim Humble was the first to extensively use this knowledge in practice, and to make it famous. In doing so he exposed himself to attack for he is not himself a medical practitioner, nor does he dance to the tune of the mass media and the pharmaceutical companies. All the people and animals MMS has already helped considered, all that matters is: He that heals, is in the right.

Chlorine dioxide is permissible for human use, including in the preparation of foodstuffs.

---

1   http://mobile.medicaltribune.de/index.php?id=446&tx_ttnews%5Btt_news%5D=17962&cHash=dc53028ed0f46edfe7791bb484618dae)

4.2 Legal aspects and the "dangers" of MMS

4.2.1 How safe is MMS?

PDF document: German Federal Institute for Risk Assessment (Bundesinstitut für Risiko-bewertung - BfR) under the search designation "MMS"

Even though MMS has been and continues to be administered successfully to thousands of humans and animals worldwide and there having been no reports of harm to the body when MMS is suitably diluted, the Internet page of the German Federal Institute for Risk Assessment (BfR) has published a PDF download document under the search word "MMS" warning against the ingestion of MMS or its active agent chlorine dioxide. Among other things it maintains:

"Thus sodium chlorite and its derivate chlorine dioxide, which is obtained through acidification, is under no account a safe nutrient ...

... In a number of European countries, and Canada and the USA as well, public health authorities have reported on the risks of 'Miracle Mineral Supplement' advising against its use. Gastrointestinal disorders of varying degrees, along with pain, nausea, vomiting and diarrhea, accompanied at times by blood pressure problems and severe fluid depletion have been observed following oral ingestion of MMS. Cases of adverse effects to health subsequent to the ingestion or intravenous injection of MMS have meanwhile been reported in Germany. In addition to nausea, vomiting and changes in general health, profound symptoms due to medical application/ utilization have become apparent. Children especially are at risk of chemical burns. The BfR (Federal Institute for Risk Assessment) strongly advises against the ingestion and the use of the product 'Miracle Mineral Supplement' (MMS)."

Dr. Hartmut Fischer, natural scientist, alternative practitioner, and author of "The DMSO Handbook" has addressed the scientific question "How poisonous is MMS." In the following chapter I would like to give a brief account of what he has discovered.

4.2.2 LD50 values

How is the evaluation by The Federal Institute for Risk Assessment to be regarded? It is easy to imagine that a mistake has obviously been made as the same institute has nowhere on its site provided a PDF document warning against the ingestion of caffeine, Diclofenac (Voltaren®), or acetylsalicylic acid (e.g., Aspirin®) to download. Anyone wishing to inform him or herself can with the aid of the relevant Wikipedia article regarding the respective substances confirm that the toxicity of these substances is conspicuously higher.

Obviously a mistake …

Definition of the term "LD50 value"

The toxicity of a substance is indicated by the LD50 value. This term derives from toxicological testing and expresses the dose in milligrams per kilogram of bodyweight required to kill half the exposed specimens, usually laboratory rats. Of course I would if I could immediately ban these animal tests, but as they have been implemented for thousands of natural and synthetic substances the hazards of ingesting a substance might as well be appraised. An institution such as the federal institute cited above normally relies on LD50 values when making its recommendations.

The toxicity of a substance is indicated by its LD50 value.

You can check this out for yourself: Search Wikipedia for the term "Chlorine dioxide." On that page, as with all (bio)chemical substances, on the right-hand side there is a long box in which at first molecular formulas and physico-chemical data are listed. At the very end of the box is "Lethal dose or concentration (LD, LC)." In this case it states:

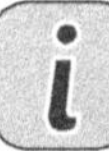

LD50 VALUE CHLORINE DIOXIDE

The LD50 value of Chlorine dioxide is 292 mg per kg bodyweight (643.749 mg/lb). This means that a person of 70 kg (154.32 lb) would need to ingest 20,000 milligram (0.705 oz) of chlorine dioxide to be critically harmed!
A (single) drop of CDS or CDSplus contains only 0.15 milligram (0.00053 oz) of chlorine dioxide. (CDS or CDSplus is the abbreviation for a ready for use solution containing 0.29% chlorine dioxide. It is the same substance as MMS, developed further; ingestion is gentler, more agreeable, and the flavor more neutral.)

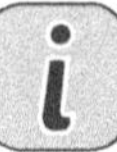

LD50 VALUE CAFFEINE

The LD50 value for caffeine is 192 mg/kg (423.29 mg/lb) for rats. It is 1.5 times less, meaning this substance is about 1.5 times more dangerous than chlorine dioxide (MMS/CDS) as a much smaller amount is required to kill the laboratory animals. A person of 70 kg (154.32 lb) need only ingest 14 g (0.00049 oz) to be subject to life threatening symptoms.

One cup of coffee in comparison to 10 drops of CDS or CDSplus

One cup of coffee contains 80 mg (0.0028 oz) of caffeine and is thus 60 times more lethal than an average dose of about 10 drops of CDS or CDSplus in a glass of water.

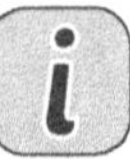

LD50 VALUES OF VOLTAREN AND ASPIRIN

Let us now search "Diclofenac" (e.g., "Voltaren®"). We learn that the LD50 value equals 62.5 mg/kg (1.377 mg/lb); apparently this is a very dangerous substance. You can proceed by searching "acetylsalicylic acid" (e.g., "Aspirin") for instance and be amazed once more, as this LD 50 value is even lower than that of chlorine dioxide. By contrast, you may be encouraged by the relative value of DMSO.

Aspirin and Voltaren compared with CDS or CDSplus

A close look at the LD50 values states that Aspirin is 1.5 times more lethal than a 0.29% solution of chlorine dioxide. Voltaren is 4 times more dangerous than a 0.29% solution of chlorine dioxide (CDS or CDSplus).

Secure handling

Handling the liquid basic substance for MMS or CDSplus (i.e., sodium chlorite solution in conjunction with a watery acid) must be done with great caution. The mixture should be diluted as quickly as possible and dosage strictly observed. The PDF document cited quite accurately states:

Please dilute mixtures promptly, and follow the directions regarding dosage.

"Direct contact with the undiluted or incorrectly prepared mixture can lead to irritation of the skin and the mucous membrane, even severe burns." Important: Do not be ambitious and overstep your individual threshold and thus induce nausea.

Good health as personal responsibility

Regarding MMS, how do things look all told? Assuming a standard volume of 0.05 ml/0.1691 fl oz per drop one would expect a drop of chlorine dioxide solution (CDS or CDS plus) to contain a maximum of 0.15 mg/0.000529 oz of CIO_2. Theoretically, a standard MMS solution (22.4% $NaCIO_2$) according to stoichiometric calculations provides a maximum of approx. 6.5 mg/0.00229 oz CIO_2 per drop assuming the chemical equivalence is taken as the basis for producing CIO_2 and an optimal reaction sequence. This is approximately forty-fold. Does this signify, the dosage instructions for the 0.29% chlorine dioxide solution (CDS or CDSplus) being valid and the classic MMS solution having reacted fully with the CIO_2, that we must dose so that 2 mL (0.0676 fl oz) of CDS (i.e., 40 drops) is equivalent to one drop of MMS?

Strength of MMS in comparison to CDS/CDSplus

So much for the theory ...

By means of various photometric laboratory measurements we know though that the activation of the standard aqueous solution of sodium chlorite (MMS) as normally conducted using acid in an open glass is less than optimal as regards the resulting amount of CIO_2.

What does this mean?

We are familiar with putting the desired number of drops of the standard 22.5% sodium chlorite solution in a glass and mixing it with the "applicable" quota of drops to bring about a proper activation. This constitutes an acid transmuting the pH value of MMS drops from highly alkaline to acid. Below pH 7 the creation of chlorine dioxide is set in motion. This is gaseous at room temperature and it begins to escape into the air immediately. Observing carefully, we can see the formation of gas bubbles in the drops. The glass is then filled with water. The solution is as a result highly dilute, after a few seconds the activation process slows considerably and is not fully discharged. Concomitantly the ClO2 that has formed in the drops is "combined" with the added water. The solubility of chlorine dioxide in water is 20 parts by volume to 1 part by volume water at 4°C (39.2 F). This would be 20 mL (0.676 fl oz) of gaseous ClO2 (approx. 50 mg/0.001763 oz) in 1 mL (0.0338 fl oz) water. At room temperature the solubility is accordingly less. In any event, ready to drink MMS solution is of a more or less yellow-green color on account of the ClO2. The two basis solutions (sodium chlorite and the activator) are nigh colorless. The light absorption of colored solutions can be analyzed with a spectrophotometer when the wavelength of light by which the colored substance absorbs photons is known. ClO2, having a light absorption coefficient of 360 nm (nanometers), lies in the ultraviolet spectral region.

Lowering the pH value releases chlorine dioxide.

Chlorine dioxide escapes as a gas during preparation.

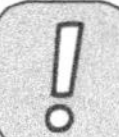

Theory and practice: Chlorine dioxide values of MMS

In practice one drop of MMS (sodium chlorite) that has been activated with one drop of 50% tartaric acid after 20 seconds of being diluted in 1000 mL (33.814 fl oz) water shows a concentration of 0.87 mg (0.003 oz) of ClO2. This is much less than the theoretical assumption of 6.5 mg (0.002 oz) ClO2 per drop of standard MMS solution!

When the decrease in the irradiated wavelengths inside a glass vessel (cuvette) containing the solution is measured with a photometer the concentration of the absorbing substance in water is deduced. How can this be explained? Firstly, as has already been detailed, a proportion of the CIO2 being generated escapes into the air before the water is poured. This is why we smell it in the room. Secondly, the transmutation of sodium chlorite into chlorine dioxide is not instantaneously accomplished with the adding of water. The drinking solution takes time to "ripen." Due to the coincident seepage into the water and diffusion caused by exposure to light no noteworthy increase in concentration can be detected with the photometer. So we are in a dilemma as a longer activation time leads to further loss of gas.

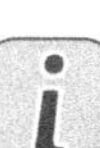

Differences in concentration of CDS or CDSplus and MMS by measure:

In practice, 1 drop of MMS equals 4 to 6 drops of CDS or CDSplus according to measurements.

LD50 VALUE of MMS

The customary amount administered is say 3 drops of MMS to one glass of water (approx. 2.61 mg/2.61 oz chlorine dioxide), far from the LD50 value (20.000 mg/0.70548 oz) that is to say by a factor of 7.663(!). According to the information contained in Wikipedia more than 22.989 drops of MMS (sodium chlorite + activator) must be imbibed (approx. 11 bottles, each containing 100 mL/3.381 fl oz sodium chlorite solution + activator) to risk death. This is not to say that it is not possible to feel unwell having taken only for instance 10 drops and/or that one may take massive amounts. Listen to your body and increase the dosage slowly, beginning with the smallest dose of 1 drop.

That the autonomous use of the chlorine dioxide solutions (CDS and CDSplus), MMS and DMSO as regards toxicity is safe in comparison to common items such as painkillers, caffeine and other substances becomes apparent, as the Federal Institute for Risk Assessment document cites reports of only minor adverse effects, gathered abroad, indicating that nothing remarkable has been detailed here in this part of the world?!

Taking this point of view, the PDF document referred to can be interpreted as special praise. Those interested in the appropriate manner in which to interpret this publication can inform themselves via this very book "MMS for Animals - A Companion Guide for the Holistic and Autonomous Treatment of Animals with MMS" and "The MMS Handbook" by Dr. med. Antje Oswald.

4.2.3 Understanding MMS

"All things are poison, and nothing is without poison, the dosage alone makes it so a thing is not a poison." said Paracelsus at the beginning of the 16th century. This applies to cooking salt (sodium chloride) as well. A tragic example from 2005 makes this clear: A four-year-old girl died after her mother, as an instructional measure, insisted her daughter eat up all the pudding into which the child had mixed two tablespoons of salt.

A sad story, unfortunately true. One gram (0.0338 oz) of salt per kilogram of body weight can kill. The pudding that the child ate contained approximately 30 g (1.0144 oz) of salt! This amount led to salt poisoning. (See: http://www.abendblatt.de/vermischtes/article753670/Tod nachSchokoPudding.html.) Nowadays, as a matter of course, we take in substances unconscious that effectively everything in excess is poison. Even water can poison us.

To determine the poisonous nature (toxicity) of substances, trials are conducted on animals under standardized conditions. All medicines, and many other substances, are tested for toxicity.

One criteria for evaluation included in such toxicity testing is the LD50 value. The LD50 value indicates the quantity of a substance capable of killing half (50%) the test objects, specific living creatures (mostly rats), under specific test conditions. It is expressed in discrete measures such as grams or milligrams or ounces, relative, as rule, to a kilogram/pound of body weight (mg/kg - mg/lb). The statistics distinguish various laboratory animals and the method of administration (oral, subcutaneous, intravenous). "LD" stands for (Median) "Lethal Dose" (Latin letalis = fatal). In this context:

LD50 value

The higher the LD50 value of a substance, the less hazardous!

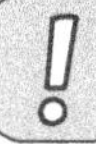

Some LD50 values: Of MMS as well as substances that are almost everyday for us

substance	product / familiar as	single dose	LD_{50} value rat oral	human body-weight of 70 kg (154,32 lb)
Dimethyl sulfoxide	DMSO	3.85 mg/a pat 0.00013 oz	14.5 mg/kg 319.6702 kg/lb	1.015.000 mg 35.803.0714 oz
Sodium chloride	common salt	a pinch	3.000 mg/kg 6.614 kg/lb	210.000 mg 7.408 oz
Ibuprofen	Nurofen	200–400 mg/ 440.924 – 881.85 oz/ tablet	636 mg/kg 1.402 mg/lb	44.520 mg 1.570 oz
Chlorine dioxide	MMS	theoretical max. 30 mg/0.00106 oz/ 5 drops	292 mg/kg 643.75 kg/lb	20.440 mg 0.721 oz
Acetylsalicylic acid (ASS)	Aspirin	500 mg/0.0176 oz/ tablet	200 mg/kg 643.75 kg/lb	14.000 mg 0.494 oz
Caffeine	Coffee	40 - 120 mg/0.0014 – 0.00423 oz/cup	192 mg/kg 423.29 kg/lb	13.440 mg 0.474 oz
Nicotine	Marlboro cigarettes	0.8 mg/0.000028 oz cigarette	50 mg/kg 110.23 kg/lb	3.500 mg 0.123 oz

Quelle: Wikipedia

What conclusions can be drawn from this information?

Even common foodstuffs such as cooking salt can be deadly in too large a dose.

To put oneself in mortal danger one would need to drink for example 10.150 one hundred mL (343.212 fl oz) bottles of DMSO, or a glass of cooking salt (in one go!), or drink 168 cups of coffee, or more than 2 bottles of activated sodium chlorite (approx. 5 drops is recommended for humans). Clearly, the dosage alone makes the poison. Even such common foodstuffs as cooking salt taken in excess can have fatal consequences, yet no package of common salt carries the warning "poison." No one would ordinarily come upon the notion of ingesting 210 g (7.407 oz) of salt. Similarly, no person, on the basis of taste alone, would consider activating and guzzling a whole bottle of MMS.

4.3 The example of a Hamburg veterinarian

Dr. Dirk Schrader is a veterinarian with his own practice in Hamburg. There he treats animals with chlorine dioxide when the need arises, preparing it himself. He has thus saved the lives of many animals when conventional medicines have brought no results.

The Hamburg Authority of Social Affairs, Family, Health and Consumer Protection, a specialist authority attached to the Hanseatic city of Hamburg, prohibited its (chlorine dioxide) production and dispensation, threatening substantial penalties. In that Dr. Schrader did not acquiesce and wanted to continue the fight to employ chlorine dioxide in his practice, I asked permission to publish the exchange of letters between him and the authority.

A Hamburg veterinarian refuses to be prevented from administering MMS.

The lawsuit was abandoned and the penalty of Euro10,000 not paid. *The public prosecutor's office was forced to drop the procedure in compliance with § 170 Abs. 2 StPO due to lack of sufficient evidence. (Update to 2nd submittal, 1.1.2018)*

"Association for Ambulatory and Clinical Therapy
26. 07. 2014

Dear Ms. XXX,
We acknowledge the prohibition of production and distribution of CDS. This is a flagrant breach of law on your part and that of your entourage. In this regard I request you and the public prosecutor's office answer the following questions:

1. In the case of an animal with a skin infection where neither the applicable antibiotics nor conventional pharmaceuticals are helpful as treatment yet we know that the chlorine dioxide lotion we prepare could unproblematically, inexpensively and without danger to the patient be effective, what then do we tell the owner of the animal?

Good outcomes treating skin infections

2. In the case of an infected wound that despite all medical endeavors gets out of hand endangering the patient's life although the sepsis could be thwarted unproblematically and inexpensively with chlorine dioxide lotion, what then do we tell the owner of the animal?

MMS et cetera: Successful in treating infected wounds, inflammation of the gums, and injury to the nail matrix

3. In the case of osteomyelitis following injury to the nail matrix and we know that amputation of the toe is unproblematically avoidable using chlorine dioxide and that diverse antibiotics would not be beneficial, what then do we tell the owner of the animal?

4. In the case of severe gingivitis (inflammation of the gums), especially common with cats, where the standard medications employed in veterinary practices are inadequate yet we know that treatment with chlorine dioxide lotion is optimal in such circumstances without putting the patient in danger, what then do we tell the owner of the animal?

5. *In the case of a septic condition such as parvovirus or colisepsis where the usual measures employed in veterinary practices bring no improvement and the patient is doomed to certain death yet we know its life could be saved with CDS infusions, what then do we tell the owner of the animal?*

6. *What do we tell the owner who brings a dog suffering malignant lymphoma and cannot afford any of the extremely expensive Vincristine treatments while we know that with the chlorine dioxide lotion we prepare the animal can be freed of this affliction, yet pursuant to your writ this is not permitted?*

Good results treating malignant lymphoma and grave, chronic ear inflammation

7. *What do we tell the customer whose dog has a grave, chronic ear inflammation that with the usual and expensive pharmaceuticals can be only partially healed while there remains the continuing danger an eardrum rupturing? Should we tell him that with chlorine dioxide lotion we could put an end to his dog's suffering, but on instruction from your agency we are not allowed?*

There are certainly more questions I could ask you and the men and women behind this scandalous writ.
Ought we tell the frustrated animal owners that the Authority for Health and Safety doesn't give a damn concerning the fate of their dog or cat? Shall we tell them that the administrative decision is based on longstanding resentments and that the whole 'club' is corrupt and morally bankrupt? Your 'club' once managed to stop the import of Arthridor, a highly effective and inexpensive osteoarthritis medication, from Israel. I was engaged in this import for many years. Suddenly this did not suit somebody in your shop and attempts were made through the AMG (German pharmaceuticals law AMG § 56a) to halt the import by any ways or means.

Obstruction of the import of Arthridor

Goodness me! Haven't you anything better to do than effect such zany schemes?

Have you and your entourage been bought up by the pharmaceutical industry? Might it be that those who do not dance to your tune are paid special attention? We will be putting this very question to the Hamburg Parliament with the aid of a party you doubtless do not like, making it public."

Further correspondence by Dr. Dirk Schrader regarding the CDS ban in his veterinary practice:

"Against German stupidity and effrontery

"Against German stupidity and effrontery
In the past year we have continued to see very sick dogs and cats. Some were mortally ill and the medications available to a modern veterinary practice could not always help. We often had the sense that the little patient has no chance if ... yes, if we do not administer the much debated chlorine dioxide. Lo and behold, most of the animals that were on the verge due to infections could survive.

That noticeably impressed us and we were able to, without blushing, encourage the owners of animals which were critically ill due to infection that chlorine dioxide, which we produce according to the rules of anorganic chemistry ourselves, puts nearly all back on their feet. It is of note that the chlorine dioxide produced was cheaper than its wrapper. A veritable sensation!

The interdiction of the preparation and administration of chlorine dioxide ordered by The Authority of Health and Consumer Protection hit us hard; and it happened as happen it must: The five-year-old Briard Vajo of XXX of Hamburg-Rahlstedt, suffering high fever, an enormous excess of leucocytes,

First death due to the ban on MMS

and fighting for his life since the weekend, died of sepsis around midday today Tuesday 05.08.2014. Every medication, including the infusion of medication, had failed.

From 03.08.2014 on we knew that something like this would come to pass; we wanted to administer chlorine dioxide but were prevented from doing so by the authorities that threatened a penalty of Euro 10,000.

Those responsible for the administrative order are:

Veterinarian Dr. XXX and his lawyer XXX
Authority of Health and Consumer Protection
Billstraße 80a 20539 Hamburg
Regarding: XXX:

Following experiences dispensing chlorine dioxide in the past we are confident that Vajo would still be alive had he undergone CD Infusion Therapy and we ask ourselves how we should proceed in the future in such cases. The seven questions were of as to be expected left unanswered. On the telephone Dr. XXX bluntly remarked: 'You can challenge the decision. You can engage a lawyer.'

Dear Colleague XXX, please take care that the sky doesn't fall on your head. You have not considered the facts concerning our chlorine dioxide case, you betray vague notions garnered from the media, which we do not wish to debate, concerning the dangers of chlorine dioxide. Correct and harmless administration in fact entails an understanding of organic chemistry, and this in turn has something to do with higher mathematics: sciences which you and your entourage are undeniably not at home with.

I expect you and your unschooled team to make contact with the dog owner and to apologize for your thoughtless actions.

I will pass on his address tomorrow. Think about the 'therapeutic freedom' (the freedom of physicians to determine therapies) guaranteed by law and the term 'emergency treatment.' Heard of these?

Dirk Schrader"

The freedom of physicians to determine therapies and emergency treatment

"The spirit that always says no …

Regarding the Administrative Order of 25.07.2014
addendum to Criminal Charge
§69Abs.1Nr.1,2and4AMG
entitles regulatory authorities to proscribe, when
1. *the requisite authorization or registration of the medicament is not presented or is suspended;*
2. *the medication or active ingredient is not prepared according to recognized pharmaceutical regulations or does not conform to the recognized pharmaceutical regulations as to quality;*
3. *when there is reasonable suspicion that the medication when administered as designated is harmful in accord with the tenable findings of medical science …"*

"Chlorine dioxide is a molecule that like cooking salt or sugar does not require authorization. Anyone can prepare it with sodium chlorite and an acid. It cannot be patented, anymore than can sodium chlorite and hydrochloric acid. The three substances are listed in neither the appendix to the AMG nor the AMK list of substances of toxicological concern.

The consequence is that chlorine dioxide neither has nor could possess the status of a medicinal product, nor can it be classi-

No authorization is required for chlorine dioxide.

fied as hazardous. On the basis of the practicability of autonomous production (§ 21, 2c AMG und § 13, 2b AMG) and its dispensation in the context of therapeutic freedom the medical application in one's own practice ought be admissible. Moreover, there is the concept of emergency treatment (§ 56a, Abs. 2 AMG) pertaining to irremediable patients or to conditions where no mainstream medicine is available that is applicable or mandatory for example.

In our practice we administer chlorine dioxide only when other available medicines offer no certainty: For instance brachycephalic surgery where so-called valve-noses are opened up by means of laser or surgery. It happened one time that a dog owner failed to attend to the operated area of the nose as agreed. She returned three weeks later, the dog no longer had a nose.

There is no substance other than chlorine dioxide that can prevent this kind of occurrence.

Positive outcomes with chronic Otitis externa

This medical sensation can also be observed when treating irremediable patients suffering chronic Otitis externa. Naturally I described this in a blog on the Internet site www.kritische-tiermedizin.de, whereupon I was accused of advertising a prohibited medication according to the AMG regulations.

Imagine that we know that chlorine dioxide is highly effective in combating malaria, or HIV infections, or even Ebola infections, and we keep this knowledge to ourselves. That would be a crime against humanity and comparable to experimental genocide.

A great deal of suffering can be avoided.

Of course chronic otitis externa with cats and dogs is no epidemic, but for animals and owners unspeakable, and in terms of veterinary expenses an existential problem. The opportunity to inform colleagues about the administration of chlorine dioxide in the form of an Internet blog was the sole means of going public. The universities would not have done so. Nevertheless, it is a sensation equal to the publication that the earth is not a disc but a sphere.

When treating 'untreatable' otitis externa with chlorine dioxide and administering it as aftercare subsequent to a nose operation in order to avert a catastrophe, and needless to say many other extremely dangerous pathogenetic developments, the oft-quoted Treatment Emergency is applicable. An actual or secondary hazard to the health of a person or animal was not and is not the occasion to concern oneself with (§21Abs.2Nr.4undAbs.2aSatz1AMG).

The contrary assertions by the responsible administrative bodies are arbitrary and unproven.
On the basis of the recognized medical procedures in our practice it is a criminal act of misrepresentation and public deception.

Meaning misrepresented.

All the same, as concerns a specialized body of the Hanseatic City of Hamburg Authority of Health and Consumer Protection, its staff members should surely have the status of 'dull-witted, mentally ill, or irresponsible.' If that is not the case then their behavior in this instance ought have legal consequences as an example of extraordinary malice and abuse of authority. I have accordingly come to believe that their high remuneration and pensions are totally unjustifiable.

Furthermore, that the author of the administrative order muddles chlorine dioxide and sodium nitrate suggests he/she has only a limited grasp of the matter.

These 'experts' write:

'The prescription, dispensation and application of the prohibited medication chlorine dioxide that is not included in any statutory instrument in accordance with § 36 oder 39 Abs. 3 Satz 1 Nr. 2, and is not a homeopathic medicine is only admissible when prepared in accordance with § 21 Abs. 2 Nr. 4 AMG pursuant to (§ 56a Abs. 1 Nr. 2 AMG).'

They are aware of the fact that chlorine dioxide requires no authorization, or not?

§ 56a Abs. 1 regulates the prescription, dispensation and application of medications by veterinarians: 'As far as necessary medical care of animals otherwise jeopardized and an actual or secondary hazard to the health of a person or animal is not to fear the veterinarian may in relation to individual animals (...)' and so on (see above).

And then they continue: 'That too does not hold true.' So the question is, in making this administrative order whether some unschooled crazy was charged from above to 'cook' the AMG (Medicinal Products Act) to prevent the dispensing of chlorine dioxide in our practice ...?

They venture to, lacking any understanding, put the following to paper:
'In our view the claims for chlorine dioxide as an effective medication and the crediting of numerous indications for its use (from AIDS through cancer to cirrhosis) are without foundation, and are for animal owners thoroughly misleading (...)'

Such claims were at no time made by me. Merits, on the basis of reports of individual experience, some of which I provided, are collected in the book by Dr. Antje Oswald (The MMS Handbook).

Efficacy is questioned without discrete studies.

They have the nerve, obviously lacking any understanding, to write further:

'It is especially misleading when therapeutic virtues, or efficacy, or efficiencies, or substance activities are attributed to medications that are not so endowed (...)'

Who are these people who proclaim such? Do they really know what they are talking about? Have they determined that chlorine dioxide is not effective treating dogs and cats suffering otitis externa for instance? Or is this an instance where halfwits who on the agency's behalf profess experience with chlorine dioxide and ... deceive?

Those responsible for the administrative order are not to be checked. They endeavor to alert The Federal Institute for Risk Assessment (BfR) to the dangers of 'MMS' maintaining and simply getting it wrong that MMS is not the same as chlorine dioxide.

The assertion that, 'chlorine dioxide affects the skin and mucous membrane, depending on the concentration, from being an irritant to being caustic' is patently false and smacks of an amateur dramatic society at The Authority of Health and Consumer Protection, out of control and without any understanding of chemistry, scrambling for arguments to make its (MMS) use impossible.

Panic is being fueled, while the recommended dilution is being disregarded.

In my letter to the authorities of 24.07.2014 I clarified that the production of chlorine dioxide in our practice resulted in an alkaline solution of pH 7.5 - 8. Damage to the skin or mucous membrane is thus not possible.

Presumably the aforementioned amateur dramatic society had not read the letter of 24.07.2014, let alone understood it. The argumentation and the bumbling concerning 'MMS' suggests criminal and diabolical intent.

MMS was never applied in our practice. Consequently, its effect on animals and humans cannot be a subject of this discussion.

Hamburg, 14.09.2014

Dirk Schrader"

The Administrative Order of July 28, 2014 forbade the production and administration of chlorine dioxide

Criminal complaint for malpractice

"I hereby file an objection to your order and simultaneously lodge a complaint at the office of the public prosecutor Hamburg against
Dr.XXX
Dr.XXX
Ms. XXX
Address

for collective malpractice and on all legal grounds file a criminal complaint.

The Facts

The rights of veterinarians

The accused lacked expertise. Discrepant to their view, a veterinarian or doctor may within the framework of Therapeutic Sovereignty (also called Therapeutic Freedom) administer in his practice substances that are not authorized according to the Medicinal Product Act to treat patients when otherwise suitable medicines are ineffective or do not suffice.

This in particular represents the legal basis for Therapeutic Emergency.

Thus it is of no matter whether the substance concerned is 'permitted' per the Medicinal Products Act or not.

The discernible harmfulness of an active substance alone can lead to the limitation of its application legally.

This is not the case with the production and administration of chlorine dioxide in our institute.

The accused allow themselves to be guided in their dealings by a superficial knowledge that they garnered through media coverage concerning a substance that can be purchased over the Internet known as MMS, the effect of which is unmistakably related to chlorine dioxide, and on that score issued a warning against its dispensation by way of The Federal Institute for Risk Assessment.

Their perception is that chlorine dioxide is prepared and administered to our patients in a comparable fashion to MMS.

The concentration is key.

This perception is false. It lacks any basis whatsoever. The plaintiff and signatory is moreover cognizant that the accused rely on extraneous rationales for their regulatory measures. Moreover, the immoderate cordiality and amity between the signatories and the government agency constituted by both the CDU and the SPD is well known. Hence this regulatory measure provides a welcome opportunity to pay off old debts.

We have long administered synthesized chlorine dioxide with 100% success, especially in regard to skin infections, without any harm to patients: Here, 20 drops of 22.5% sodium chlorite solution is mixed with 20 drops of 3.5% hydrochloric acid for exactly 1 minute and diluted in 60 mL (2.0288 fl oz) tap water. Mindful of the poisonous nature of the gases discharged, the preparation is conducted beneath ventilators, and/or before an open window.

"... without any harm to patients"

Dabbing the infected areas of skin with this solution (pretreatment with a 50% DMSO solution enables a more intensive action) results in the immediate elimination of all microorganisms within reach. As a precaution this process is repeated a number of times.

Allergy related skin inflammations are, where applicable, treated in parallel with cortisone and/or antihistamines.

Example of application: Infection of the airways

In cases of infections of the airways or the gastro-intestinal tract

We bring 1 - 2 drops of 22.5% sodium chlorite solution with 1 - 2 drops of 3.5% hydrochloric acid solution together for exactly 1 minute (a common shot glass works best), 2 - 5 mL (0.067 - 0.169 fl oz) tap water is then added; draw the diluted mixture back into the syringe and dispense this directly into the animal's mouth (ideally to the side, into the cheek pouch). This treatment takes place following the intake of food (never on an empty stomach!), twice daily in dramatic situations. Here too, no harm to patients has ever been observed. Therapy resistant infections such as parvovirus or colisepsis are treated with this infusion. As a matter of interest we have been able to halt seven cases of malignant lymphoma in dogs with this oral method since 2013.

To assist with the following descriptions by Dr. Hartmut Fischer, Lauterbach, a glossary is indispensable.

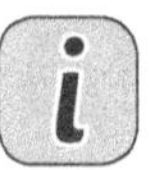

Definitions: Sodium chlorite and Chlorine dioxide

Sodium chlorite

... is a crystalline solid, which is directly formed by the conversion of chlorine dioxide with caustic soda/sodium hydroxide due to disproportionation or the addition

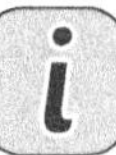

Continuation: Sodium chlorite and chlorine dioxide

of hydrogen peroxide. Toxicity: 165 mg/kg - 1 / 363.762 mg/lb (LD50 Rat, oral).

Chlorine dioxide

ClO2 is released when it is acidified in an aqueous solution or is displaced with chlorine. It is gaseous at room temperature with a maximum absorption of approx. 355 nm, and exhibits a yellow-green color. Toxicity: 292 mg/kg - 1 / 643.749 mg/lb - 1 (LD50 Rat, oral). The scientific literature regarding ClO2 shows circa 1200 entries on the search portal SiFinder, which brings fundamental research as well as applications in industry and medicine together. Disintegration of chlorine dioxide is accelerated by exposure to light and various products such as chlorite and chlorate. It dissolves readily in water

Toxicity in comparison: Diclofenac (Voltaren) 62.5 mg/kg - 1 /1.377,889 - 1 mg/lb (LD50 Rat, oral), acetylsalicylic acid (Aspirin) 200 mg/kg - 1 / 440.924 mg/lb (LD50 Rat, oral); both are more toxic than chlorine dioxide. MMS, on the other hand, is an artificial word that is neither a specific substance definition nor a registered product name/trademark. In general it designates an aqueous mix of sodium chlorite and an anorganic or organic acid with a pH value significantly below 7. Aqueous solutions composed of sodium chlorite and acids that indicate a pH value >7 go through an extended dynamic constituting a number of intermediate stages; are free of chlorine dioxide as well. One speaks of ClO2 in statu nascendi (from the Latin: in the state of being born).

Voltaren and Aspirin are more toxic than chlorine dioxide

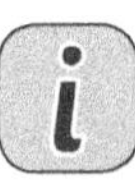

Neither chlorine dioxide nor sodium chlorite appears in the AMG or AMK list of substances of concern. This means that neither has the status of a medicinal product nor is it classified as being of concern. On the strength of autonomous production (§ 21, 2c AMG und § 13, 2b AMG) and administration in the framework of Therapeutic Freedom, medical use in one's own practice ought be possible in general. In addition, there is the term Treatment Emergency (§ 56a, Abs. 2 AMG) that applies when for instance treating so-called irremediable patients or illnesses for which no mainstream medications are available. Needless to say, know-how, rigor, provision of patient education, et cetera come to the fore - not in question in my case."

"Inappropriate application, over dosage, et cetera by therapists and lay people is certainly possible, and does happen, but this observation applies, without exception to every widely administered (active) substance and every officially approved medicinal product. That the dose makes the poison is well known to be the case for even cooking salt.

Chlorine dioxide is categorized as an oxidizing agent in biochemistry; included are substances that transfer oxygen atoms, or, owing to their electronegativity, accept negative elementary charges in the form of electrodes, or effect both actions concurrently. A wide range of these substances is employed in medicine and therapy - ozone, hydrogen peroxide, potassium permanganate, artesunate (an organic peroxide), and hypochlorite included. With respect to sodium chlorite and chlorine dioxide, hydrogen peroxide and hypochlorite especially, it has been acknowledged in the realm of clinical immunology for de-

cades (and at times the Nobel Prize has been awarded) that in cases of a reaction to fever with infections and cancer, etcetera, and also physiologically in humans and animals, cells appear i.e., are produced. Oxidative active agents possess vital advantages: Microorganisms cannot develop resistance; we can therefore assure 'Evolution' of a gratifying providence.

Inversely, human and animal cells inherently tolerate a certain measure of oxidative substances, whilst microorganisms or miscellaneous antigens are destroyed with appreciably lesser concentrations. *That is why ozone for instance can be infused despite its counting as the strongest poison for organic matter. As with every oxidant including chlorine dioxide it is paramount that both the supportable and effective dose where this can take place be identified.*
Many, quantitatively significant applications are indicated for chlorine dioxide, among them the treatment of drinking water in accordance with regulations of the same name, or the treatment of processed water in the drink, milk and food industries. This on the basis of the ability of chlorine dioxide to kill practically all viruses, bacteria, spores, mildews, and even prions![1] Only the notoriously resistant microbacteria are somewhat impervious to CLO2.

In the year 2000 it was already established in toxicological tests that: ... higher organisms are relatively unaffected when chlorine dioxide is orally ingested. **For instance, in a study where ten healthy men were administered 24 mg/0,000846 oz (of chlorine dioxide in a Liter of water, that is to say 2.5 mg (0.000882 oz) chlorite in 500 mL (16.90 fl oz) of water, no negative changes were observed.[2]**

Bacteria cannot develop resistance to chlorine dioxide.

Higher organisms are relatively non-sensitive to chlorine dioxide.

---

1   Seymour Stanton Block: Disinfection, sterilization and preservation December 15, 2000, p. 215 f. .

2   Toxicological Review regarding chlorine dioxide and chlorite by the U.S. Environmental Protection Agency (EPA), Washington D.C., September 2000.

Likewise, the EFSA (European Food Safety Authority) determined: '... moreover, despite a long history of utilization, there is no public data to suggest that the use of chlorine dioxide leads to increased bacterial tolerance against chlorine dioxide or increased resistance to therapeutic antibiotics and antimicrobial agents.' The Federal Institute for Risk Assessment expressed the view that chicken meat treated with chlorine dioxide is not hazardous to health of the consumer and in terms of asepsis has advantages.'"

"Patents relating to Chlorine dioxide

Chlorine dioxide has long been the subject of medical research and application, which is evidenced by the numerous patent specifications literature. Examples are:

US 4.03 5,$^{483}/_{12}$ .07.1977 for the use of sodium chlorite as a non-poisonous Antiseptic '... beneficial when treating burns and other wounds and treating infections without the natural regeneration process being interfered with ...'

US 2,70 1,$^{781}/_{08}$. 02.1955 Commercial exploitation of an antiseptic solution for general clinical use.

US 5,01 9,$^{402}/_{28}$. 05.1991 Firm of Alcide for the commercialization of a product with chlorine dioxide as disinfectant for blood and conserved blood. Alcide (a mixture of sodium chloride and lactic acid) can currently be found in the ECOLAB portfolio of products under the name 'LD,' and is other than that the only preparation to be in accordance with toxicological expert evaluation to be ClO_2.

US 5,83 0,$^{511}/_{03}$. 11.1998 for the commercialization of a product, the ingredient also being sodium chlorite, for stimulation of the

Stimulation of the immune system
Reduced mortality
Reduced dependence on antibiotics
Improvement in the state of health of animals

immune system. Issued to the firm of Bioxy Inc. to be used as feed a supplement for animals, leading to reduced mortality, reduced excretion of nitrogen, reduced dependence on antibiotics and vaccinations, and improvement of the state of health of animals.

US 5,85 5,$^{922}/_{05}$. 01.1999, issued to the concern BioCide International for the commercialization of a product for therapeutic treatment of chronic wounds healing insufficiently or not scarring over, and other skin ailments.

US 6,09 9,$^{855}/_{08}$. 08.2000 immunity stimulant for animals, issued to the firm Bioxy Inc.

US 4,29 6,$^{102}/_{20}$. 10.1981 for the commercialization of a product to combat amebic dysentery in humans via the oral dispensation of chlorine dioxide. Patent issued to Felipe Lazo, Mexico City.

US 6,25 1, 372 B$^{1}/_{26}$. 06.2001 issued to Procter & Gamble for the commercialization of a product to prevent bad breath.

Combats bad breath

S 4,85 1,$^{222}/_{25}$. 07.1989, issued to the firm Oxo for the commercialization of a product for the regeneration of bone marrow.

Regeneration of the bone marrow

US 4,73 7, $^{307}/_{02}$. 04.1988 for the commercialization of a product to combat bacteria, funguses, and viruses vis à vis skin ailments.

Skin ailments and burns

US 5,25 2,$^{343}/_{02}$. 03.1982 issued to Felipe Lazo of Mexico for the commercialization of a medication to treat burns to the skin.

US 5,25 2,$^{343}/_{12}$. 10.1993 issued to the firm Alcide for the commercialization of a product for the prevention and treatment of bacterial infections, especially mastitis, where up to 1000 ppm chlorine dioxide is administrated.

Mastitis

EP 2508474 A1/30. 03.2012 plus cross references, Fa. Wacker Chemie, chlorine dioxide stabilized by alpha-ayclodextrin as a molecular container, proposed for adhesive plaster among other purposes. In the description, and most notably, the selectivity of ClO_2 in comparison with other oxidants is emphasized which makes its application to human and animal tissue inevitable.

Dioxychlor

Naturally, patents are not evidence of efficacy as regards elicitation of clinical data. Such attestation can be found in the literature as ClO_2, going by the Anglo-Saxon name Dioxychlor, was already in use with demonstrable success in the 1980s, primarily by doctors at the famed Mayo clinics, having been developed and generally applied as a solution for infusion for all kinds of maladies. Relevant reports can be examined via medical faculties in the USA. From toxicological works under Application of the Mixture of Sodium Chlorite and Lactic Acid one learns:
'... it is excellent for Herpes, nail fungus (onychomycosis), warts, and the treatment of infective burns. The active ingredients in this compound are sodium chlorite and lactic acid. It has shown itself to be extremely effective, especially with long-established, chronic sicknesses where no other product is of assistance.' [1]

Further medico-scientific evidence regarding efficacy and suitable chlorine dioxide preparations in sensible doses can be researched by all and sundry.

The present-day, emotionally driven and unjust 'witch hunt' against the oxidant commonly employed for decades is,

---

1   M. S. AbdelRahman, S. E. Gerges and H. Alliger, Toxicity af Alcide, Journal of applied Toxicology, Vol. 2, No. 3, S. 160, 1982.

considered in this light, not objectively comprehensible. Only a marked absence of basic scientific understanding, very likely under the influence of jealous colleagues, or media representatives hungry for headlines, could have precipitated the arraignment and threat of punishment. This typifies the medical-historical Semmelweis Reflex that sad to say often comes into play subsequent to apposite research projects that have improved therapeutic practices, and that can only be implemented fifty years later due to obstruction by institutional powers - I very much hope this will not be the case here. It is plain and simply a matter of the actuality of Therapeutic Freedom in Medicine, substantiated through millennia, without which not a single accomplishment of modern medicine would have been possible.

I thank Dr. Hartmut Fischer for his making his boilerplate texts available to me.

Dirk Schrader, ltd TA (senior Veterinarian)"

Semmelweis-Reflex

The lawsuit was abandoned and the penalty of Euro10,000 not paid. *The public prosecutor's office was forced to drop the procedure in compliance with § 170 Abs. 2 StPO due to lack of sufficient evidence. (Update to 2nd submittal, 1.1.2018)*

4.4 Jim Humble

When I first met Jim Humble in the flesh he was, I believe, eighty-one-years young. I met a man in ripe old age with plans for the future - I would say another eighty years. He radiated geniality and warmth.

He radiates geniality and warmth…

Much has been written about Jim Humble and the history of MMS. For those who perhaps have come into contact with MMS for the fist time, here is a short abstract:

Jim Humble

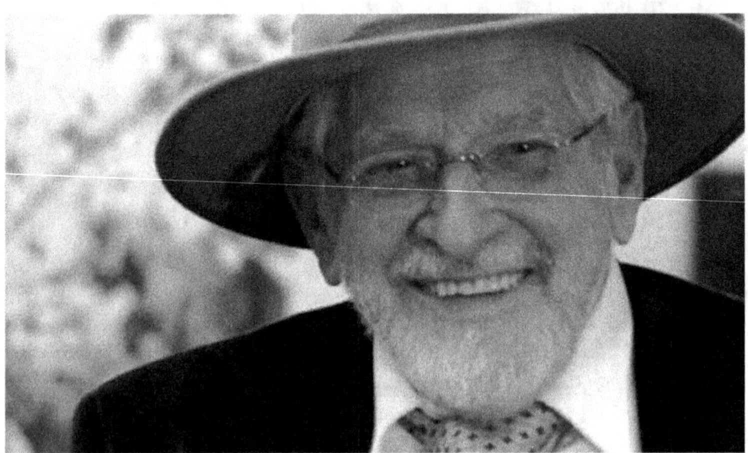

Jim Humble - Originator of "MMS"

Jim Humble was a gold miner, and in this capacity he travelled to Guyana in1996 to search for gold in the jungles of South America. Being aware, on account of previous travel experience, of the risks of using water, from rivers for instance, he brought stabilized oxygen with him. Two of his crew came down with malaria deep in the jungle. He dispatched some men to another mine to ask for help or medicines, but that might have required six days. Waiting could have had grievous consequences in that malaria often ends in death. (Worldwide, malaria kills 1.2 million people yearly.) Radio communication is not viable in the jungle, so it was a question of waiting. Jim Humble had an idea out of the blue. He thought to himself that the human body consists of 70% water and that it must be feasible to sterilize this water in the body. Having stabilized oxygen on hand, he asked the sick men whether they wished to imbibe this "Health Drink" as he called it. They agreed, and four hours later they were doing so well that they were able to partake of the evening meal. When on the following day more men came down with malaria they were instantly proffered the "Health Drink" - it helped again.

Later on, in 1997, when Jim Humble was back home, he research further out of his own interest. He wanted to know what stabilized oxygen really consisted of as this

Continuation: Jim Humble - Originator of "MMS"

was not indicated on the packaging. Since he lacked the means and knowledge of a chemist it took rather a long time. Nevertheless, he found out that oxygen was not the grounds for the healing.

But first things first: Initially he experimented with stabilized oxygen and vinegar in a glass of water. When he allowed this glass to stand for 24 hours it smelled distinctly of chlorine. The whole process and the preparation took too long, though, to make sense in everyday practice. What was the basis for this reaction? Was the healing related somehow to the chlorine?

Stabilized oxygen is stable due to its being a strong base. When combined with water the base value sinks, the ions in the drops become unstable and chlorine is, as he first believed, freed. So how could the reaction be speeded up? He researched further with various acids and found that 5% acetic acid, an organic acid, functioned best in lowering the base value. After long research he ultimately ascertained that the ingredient of stabilized oxygen is: Sodium chlorite or $NaClO_2$.

Why then was it called "stabilized oxygen"? Because the sodium chloride has stably bonded oxygen to itself (thereby becoming sodium chlorite). First with the addition of an acid is the oxygen that has bonded with chlorine to become chlorine dioxide released; the chlorine atom bonds with sodium becoming sodium chloride (cooking salt). Chlorine dioxide is thus biodegradable.

The mix tasting execrable, he tried out diverse juices and decided on apple juice without added vitamin C. Why without vitamin C? The action of chlorine dioxide has as its basis oxidation and artificial vitamin C is a strong antioxidant; allow an interval of at least four hours when ingesting vitamin C in a high dose.

It was clear to Humble that a chemist probably would have found this all out in half an hour. Many would think that this sounds like salt. Table salt too has the formula $NaCl$ and is called "sodium chloride." The fine and meaningful difference is in the last letter.

Sodium chlorite solution is highly alkaline (basic), the opposite to sour. Sodium chlorite solution when neutralized becomes unstable, does not release oxygen but

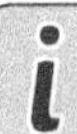

Continuation: Jim Humble – Originator of "MMS"

chlorine dioxide. With more testing Jim Humble discovered that chlorine dioxide is the oxidant and not the oxygen.

Over time Jim Humble built contacts with Africa where he treated thousands for malaria.

MMS stands for "Miracle Mineral Supplement." MMS did not receive approval as a medication in Africa either, therefore he designated it as "Supplement," i.e., dietary supplement, though it is not, with the aim of obtaining certification. The word "Miracle" was ultimately dropped as many people were uncomfortable with using a "Wonder Drug," the whole terrain having negative (media-driven) connotations. Still, miracles happen again and again with this substance. For a number of years the acronym "MMS" has officially stood for "Master Mineral Solution."

Jim Humble, having by his own account freed many thousands of people in Africa from malaria thanks to MMS, approached the WHO. The response from the authorities was lapidary: Without any in depth investigation, it was communicated that the substance did not function with mice, hence for them the matter was concluded.

Following many set backs MMS finally came into currency, and Jim wished to communicate this to all. The book "MMS - Breakthrough" came into being; there is a section you can, if you wish, download free of charge in the Internet. How to prepare the solution is no secret either: Anyone who wants to, and is able to access the ingredients, can do so, can prepare it at a very reasonable price themselves.

This is a short summary of Jim Humble's story, which I have in part retold in his own words, quoting from the book "MMS – Breakthrough." There, you can read the whole story and of the challenges involved.

The events depicted have the hallmarks of a present-day witchhunt. Many others who have discovered something sensational or especially beneficial have suffered similar fates; as an example one could read in the May 2014 issue of the VDT newspaper (Verband Deutscher Tierheilpraktiker - Association of German Alternative Practitioners for Animals):

"Dr. Glenn Warner, successful holistic doctor, treated thousands of cancer patients, healing more than a thousand. His aim was to comprehend the sickness, build up the immune system, and to heal. A feature of his treatment was healthy nutrition. His office was raided, his license revoked.
Dr. Max Gerson who had success employing nutrition therapy with cancer sufferers fled to Mexico in order to practice there as his professional life in the USA was made hell."

"Threat" owing to healthy nutrition

These are just two of many examples. This happens not just in America but overall - in Germany as well, sadly. Presently such a controversy, as you may have already read, involving a Hamburg veterinary practice, is under way. In my opinion we can do without a "funeral pyre" or a "witch-hunt." For myself too, I wish for self-determination in relation to therapy and medication. I am gratified working towards this, and support autonomous treatment as far I am able.

Regarding me personally, I wish to make this clear: I have no association with Scientology or any sect as is persistently insinuated - and thematized in the media - in reference to MMS and people identified with it. In my view, personal matters have nothing to do with the substance. Are films by a Tom Cruise or a Will Smith less successful on account of their engagement with a sect? I often ask myself what is actually at issue: MMS, or Jim Humble, or the play of power? Each to their own opinion.

Scientology

MMS has found its place in the world, is unstoppable. So far approximately one million books on this theme have been sold worldwide in about twenty languages thanks to those such as Dr. Andreas Kalcker with his new CDS (chlorine dioxide solution) who are fascinated by the substance and work on research and further development.

1 million MMS books sold in over 20 languages

It is of course important to decide on one's own volition whether or not to use this medicine with one's animals. You will never hear from me that you must, or that it is the only course of action. For every situation there are many possibilities; this one may be good for the health of your animals.

4.5 Types of MMS

MMS as appellation is prohibited, look for Sodium Chlorite and Activator

As mentioned in the early chapters MMS is a designation invented by Jim Humble. When I first used MMS I recall there was a sticker referring to MMS and Jim Humble on the bottles of sodium chlorite and citric acid., This is now regrettably prohibited.

A woman who has known MMS for years recently asked me why MMS is no longer available. As she was enthusiastic about the substance, and Jim Humble as well, she could not comprehend this and all the new products such as CDSplus; she found it all to be confusing.

I hope with this chapter to bring some clarity in respect to the various forms of MMS.

4.5.1 MMS or MMS 1

The original MMS consisted of two components: Sodium chlorite and 10% citric acid. Needless to say, this is still on the market, though the evolution continues through the efforts of Jim Humble, Andreas Kalcker and many other wonderful people.

The classic MMS still exists, though no longer under this name. It is identifiable as a bottle of 22.5% Sodium Chlorite Solution and a bottle of Activator: Citric acid, tartaric acid, hydrochloric acid, or lactic acid. It is still in common use as it is very effective and has a long shelf life. The downside relative to CDS or CDS-plus is the intense odor and taste.

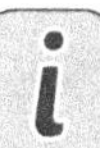

Distinctive features when taking MMS

When taking MMS (activated with an acid and diluted in water) note that a second activation transpires due to the gastric acids. Therefore a slow and careful build up is critical! The activation as a result of the body's own juices can be used to one's advantage in that the acid can be reduced, e.g., 2 drops of sodium chlorite and 1 drop of acid, or the acid can be eliminated. Sodium chlorite then reacts first in the areas of the body where that are acid or overly acid. In this way the effect is not premature, it aids with bacteria in situ through oxidation, and simultaneously alters the balance from sour to alkaline. Most of the sicknesses attendant to civilization arise due to over acidification (acidosis). The water in the body "tips," in effect stagnating, and in this setting bacteria, viruses, and cancers are encouraged. Cancer in fact requires an acid environment to develop.

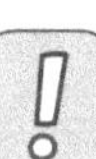

Chlorine dioxide attaches, so to say, to the red blood cells and by this means courses throughout the body. It kills viruses and bacteria on contact; they are combusted and then excreted through the normal bodily processes. It was once explained to me in this way: The mechanism can be described as electrical flashes that strike the bacteria and the like incinerating them as though with an electrical charge. This is certainly oversimplification; for a detailed, scientific expositions, and explanations see the Bibliography at the end of the book.

4.5.2 Chlorine dioxide solution (CDS)

CDS is composed of the same active ingredients as MMS (chlorine dioxide), the difference being that with CDS the chlorine dioxide is processed in such a way that it is appreciably more pleasant to imbibe and administer.

The advantages of CDS in detail:

a) Only one bottle needs be constituted instead of two.

b) The solution is already prepared; no more substances must be brought together to react.

c) The strong odor is gone as no chemical reaction takes place.

d) The flavor is appreciably friendlier and milder.

e) It is possible to administer CDS intramuscularly to animals.

f) CDS is considerably more agreeable and gentler.

(Quoted from Dr. Antje Oswald, "The MMS Handbook." See: Bibliography.)

Use either CDS/CDSplus or MMS with hydrochloric acid

Andreas Kalcker, a biophysicist, filmmaker, and author developed this solution when a calf-breeder requested a special solution. The problem was that for the breeding of calves much medicine is needed and he could no longer afford it. Due to stomach issues MMS could not be administered. After some

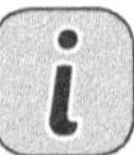

Comparison of MMS to CDS

Theoretically the approximate values are:

The pH of MMS lies between 2.5 - 3 and is thus designated acid. The pH of CDS lies between 5.5 - 7 and is thus almost neutral.

An important difference is the shelf life. MMS can be stored for years. CDS keeps for only weeks or months (preferably in darkness, in the refrigerator). **CDSplus when not activated can be stored for a number of years.** Following activation the shelf life is weeks or months according to how it is stored and frequency of use.

MMS is four times stronger than 0.29% chlorine dioxide solution.

CDS is for this reason milder, and unlike MMS is normally not accompanied by diarrhea and vomiting with higher dosages.

time it was established that this distress was caused by the strong acid employed as an activator and not the MMS itself. Combining sodium chlorite with a low concentration of hydrochloric acid (approx. 5%), or sodium chlorite without acid solved this problem. In the end this situation brought positive change.

Chlorine dioxide is, like MMS, distilled by means of a time-honored process employing two components whereby the gas given off binds with cooled water, resulting in a 0.29% pure chlorine dioxide solution. This should be stored in the refrigerator.

4.5.3 CDSplus

CDSplus is a further development of CDS, is an, so to say, "always fresh" CDS. The biggest problem as regards CDS, its shelf life, has been resolved. The package contains a sachet of activator. The powder is tipped into the bottle on demand, the bottle is then shaken and the CDSplus allowed to stand for four hours at room temperature. The 0.29% solution in now ready for use and can be administrated in the same way as the familiar CDS. It should then be stored in the refrigerator. The advantage of CDSplus is that it keeps for many years, ready to be activated when needed, and then just the one time for the whole bottle. It then possesses the same positive, mild and agreeable attributes as regular CDS.

CDSplus: The first long lasting and standardized chlorine dioxide solution

Compraison between CDS and CDSplus

compraison	CDS	CDSplus
shelf life	weeks/months	years/following activation like CDS
vacation	difficult, due to cooling	simple, due to on-site activation

CDSplus lasts longer.

4.5.4 Gefeu solution

Better reaction Yet another option is the Gefeu solution whereby the pure gas
using a syringe is used in conjunction with activated MMS. The activation
takes place entirely in the syringe. The acid converts more
thoroughly when the activation transpires in the syringe and
the Gefeu solution is milder to the taste than the MMS mixture. Another advantage is that the solution must be dispensed
only three times daily as opposed to hourly as is often required
with CDS. It too, is very effective. Further, it has a long shelf
life. Refrigerated it retains full potency for a year according to
a therapist. Gefeu solution is not to be purchased as such, but
can and must be prepared on the spot.
Gefeu solution can be prepared oneself. Instructions are to be
found in Chapter 5.5.

What sets Gefeu solution apart is that the process is a closed-cir-
cle, contact with the air being limited, and only when the reaction is complete is it administered. The acid content is therefore
significantly less, and the solution diluted in water is more
agreeable than MMS.

Advantage: The advantage of Gefeu solution is that due to the special meth-
Less acid od of preparation less acid is used while as much chlorine dioxide as possible is produced. To keep activation time within
practicable limits the thinning in water is first carried out when
activation is fully complete.

The Gefeu solution therefore always comprises almost exactly
1% (= 10.000 ppm) concentration of chlorine dioxide. Measurements indicate that this is nevertheless a theoretical value: Gefeu solution is in practice around seven times weaker than MMS,
meaning it is well-nigh the same potency as CDS and CDSplus.

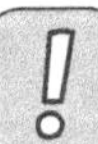

1 drop of MMS corresponds to approx. 7 drops of Gefeu solution.

4.5.5 MMS Globules

As with other homeopathic globules, MMS globules are primed on an energetic plane. MMS and CDS Energy globules are ethereally informed sources of energy for humans who are interested in energetic medicine. In my experience, they are borne by the human body and deliver their information. We have dispensed homeopathic globules to animals orally. The responses differed markedly, and with some animals it was necessary to provide reinforcement with CDS. Energy globules can be obtained from Dr. Antje Oswald (http://shop.informierteglobuli.de).
If there are any new developments or discoveries I will post these and potential suppliers on my website under www.mobile-tierheil praxismonika.de.

Energetic action

4.5.6 MMS 2

MMS 2 generally comes in the form of capsules. These capsules contain calcium hypochlorite powder. For humans two glasses of water should be ingested first, the capsule swallowed, and lastly another glass of water taken in. As this is extremely difficult, if not impossible, I advise against this with animals. When there is too little liquid the capsule can break open in the esophagus and mix with the water producing hypochlorous acid which is highly caustic. Aside from that, calcium hypochlorite lacks the positive attributes of an oxidant. In that it is generally difficult to dispense I advise against it. MMS 2 is better suited to humans suffering severe illness as a supplement to MMS to bolster efficacy.

MMS 2 must be imbibed with plenty of water.

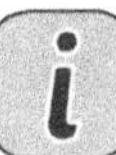

Differences between MMS and MMS 2

MMS and MMS 2 are two different compounds.

MMS is sodium chlorite that is bonded with an activator in the form of an acid (citric acid, hydrochloric acid et cetera), resulting in chlorine dioxide. MMS 2 is calcium hypochlorite, water is added as the activator = hypochlorous acid.

MMS 2 is combined with MMS when treating severe ailments such as cancer.

MMS 2 should not be administered on its own, but in combination with MMS. MMS 2 is NOT A SUBSTITUTE FOR MMS!

MMS 2 is not recommended for animals: It is available in the form of capsules which must be taken in with at least 300 mL (10.144 fl oz) of water then transported to the stomach where the capsule is broken down by the gastric juices and activated. When not enough water is imbibed the capsule remains in the throat for too long, which can lead to chemical burns. Exercise caution and love with your animals when dispensing MMS and CDS - this will suffice.

4.5.6 Tabular overview of MMS varieties

Substance	Activation	Advantage	Disadvantage	Bear in mind
MMS 1	preparation on the spot, activation when required	most effective of all; simple administration; has proved itself in a multitude of situations over the years; keeps for years	must be activated; produces a very strong odor; tastes strongly of chlorine; low palatability	caustic following activation, must be diluted in water
CDS	pre-prepared solution, activation not required	for immediate use; taste and palatability friendly and mild due to the method of production	short self life, must be stored in the refrigerator; not as strong as MMS 1	potential loss of chlorine dioxide solution when in storage and transported; must be thinned in water
CDSplus	activation when required, and then only one time for the whole bottle	keeps for years before activation; following activation and stored cool for weeks or months. Ideal as a standardized and fresh chlorine dioxide solution to have on hand. Taste and palatability friendly and mild	potency lies between CDS and MMS. Can be understood as a strong CDS	relatively resistant to heat and light, can accordingly be taken along on foreign journeys. Must be diluted in water
Gefeu	activation necessary	contains much gaseous chlorine dioxide - taste and agreeability somewhat friendlier than MMS; keeps in refrigerator for months	must be prepared oneself - strength can vary according to preparation and raw materials; not as strong as MMS 1	must be diluted in water
MMS 2	offered in capsules consisting of calcium hypochlorite; activated with water	employed to counter diseases such as cancer; in combination with MMS 1 is administered to humans	must be imbibed with plenty of water, otherwise the capsule breaks open in the esophagus; is activated by the water and a very caustic hypochlorous acid is produced	not suitable for animals; the ingredients are different than those of MMS

5

MMS –
The Practical Section

5.1 How do I activate MMS?

Preparing MMS solution

You have obtained the two components Sodium chlorite and acid beforehand. These two bottles now stand in your house. What to do with them and what should you be aware of?

Preparing a MMS solution

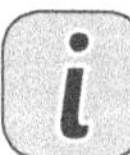

Materials for the preparation of the MMS solution:

- Bottle Sodium chlorite
- Bottle acid
- 1 clean and dry glass

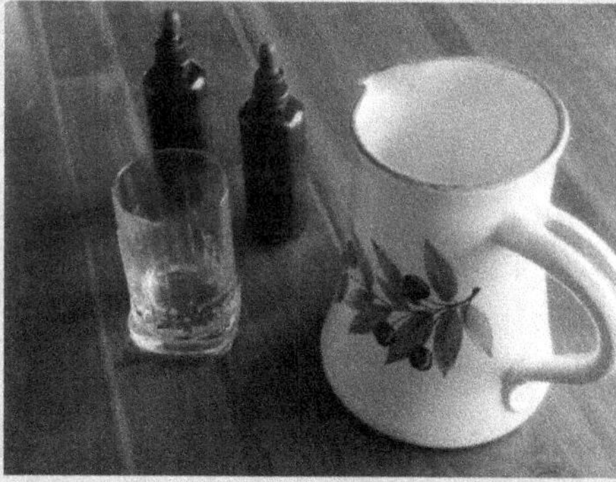

First drip the required drops, e.g., 2 drops of sodium chlorite into the glass. Add the acid. In the illustration 2 drops of 50% citric acid is used. It is important to jiggle the glass so that the two liquids mix. Wait 30 to 45 seconds (mix ratio and activation times of various acids are to found in Chapter 6). During this procedure (activation) we can observe how the color changes. Next we dilute the mixture with the applicable amount of water (100 mL/3.381 fl oz in this case). This fluid can be utilized straight away.

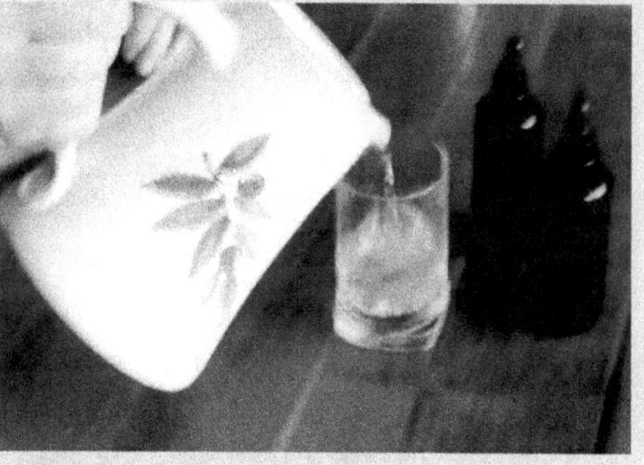

When activating MMS it is important to adhere to the following: Where possible work close to an open window or with an extractor hood running. Avoid directly breathing in the fumes! Avoid spraying the undiluted, activated liquid on the skin or clothing, as it is caustic in this state!

5.2 Quick and simple preparation of CDS in small amounts according to Dr. Hartmut Fischer

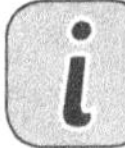

Preparing CDS in small amounts[1]

Materials for the quick preparation of CDS:

- Safety goggles
- Syringe, approx. 30 mL (1.014 fl oz) or more
- Tubing, approx. 70 mm (2.75 in.) or better 40 cm (15.75 in.) long hosing that fits over the syringe nozzle
- Sodium chlorite 22.5 %
- Acid, e.g., hydrochloric 5 - 10 % or another acid (but not lactic acid as the production of gas is slow)
- Glass of water

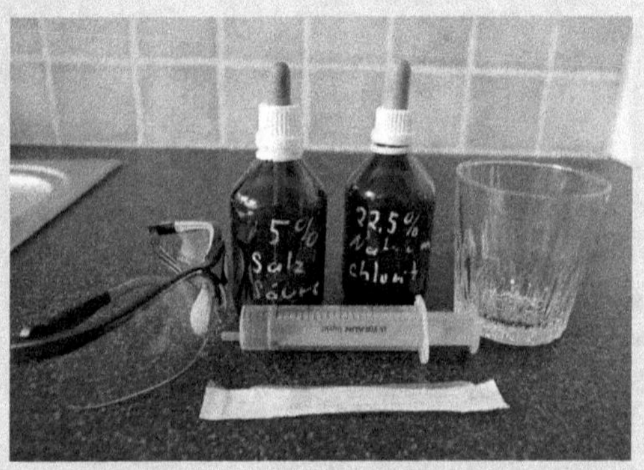

[1] Of course one can buy pre-prepared CDS or CDSplus. That is always the simplest way out. Preparing the solution oneself is most likely cheaper and ensures that it is fresh. This method is the royal road to preparing high-purity chlorine dioxide oneself (perhaps even for infusion), as it entails a process of distillation whereby only the pure active ingredient remains.

1

First please put on the protective goggles and then fill the glass with water.

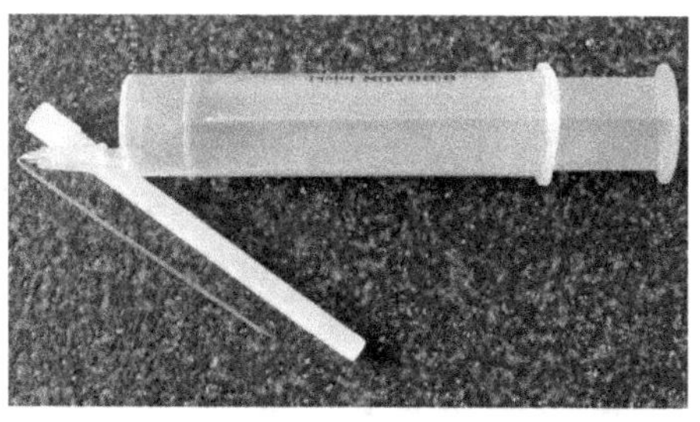

Hold the syringe at right angles with the needle and protective sleeve (the plastic sheath enclosing the needle) facing up. Pull the sleeve upwards about 4 mm (0.157 in.) and carefully bend the needle down at the base of the sleeve approx. 150 degrees (see picture). Alternatively, attach a 40 cm (15.75 in.) long tube onto the nozzle of the syringe - the needle is no longer necessary - any danger of injury from the needle is thus averted.

2

Now pull the plunger out of the syringe and hold the syringe opening facing up. Hold the syringe at a gentle angle so that the liquid will not run out.

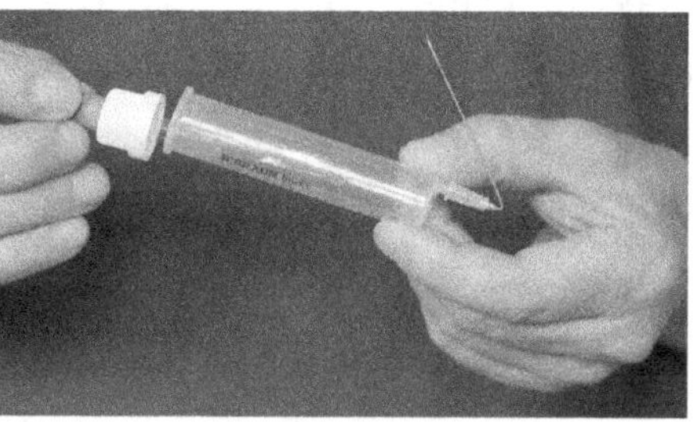

Drip five drops of sodium chlorite into the syringe followed by five drops of acid. The sodium chlorite should not yet bind with the acid.

3

Slide the plunger just a few millimeters (0.2 in.) into the syringe and then angle the plunger downwards.

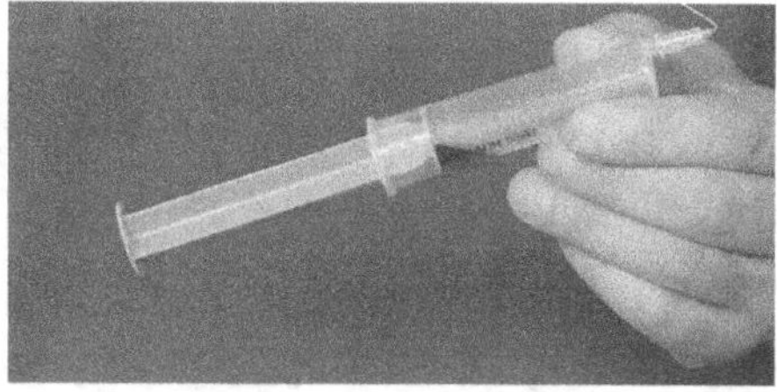

Gently rotate the syringe causing the sodium chlorite and acid to make contact and thus react, the end product being chlorine dioxide. You will recognize this when you see the air pocket in the syringe turn yellow due to the chlorine dioxide gas.

4

First when the gas in syringe exhibits a distinctly yellow color dip the needle into the water and with gentle pressure squirt the chlorine dioxide gas into the water.

Take note! Take care to squirt only gas into the water and not the reacting fluid!

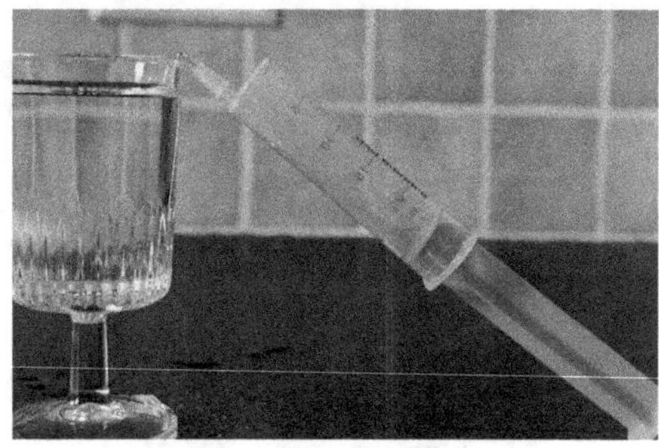

5

Now take the syringe out of the glass of water, hold it with the plunger inclined downward, carefully draw air into the syringe again, wait until the syringe fills with yellow chlorine dioxide gas, and squeeze this into the glass once again.

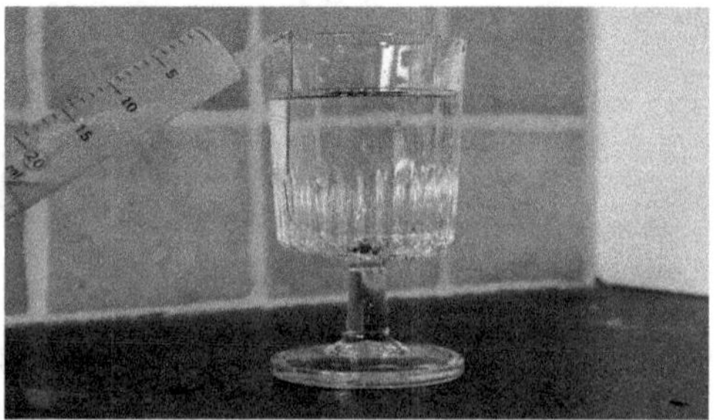

6

This procedure can be repeated so long as the yellowish chlorine dioxide gas keeps building.

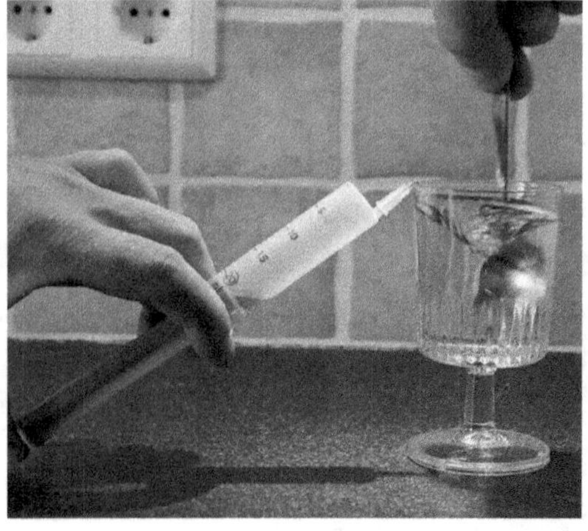

Now you have a pure and perfectly distilled chlorine dioxide solution untainted by admixtures of impurities. As regards the potency, it is not possible to state this accurately as this is contingent on a multitude of factors. In dealing with CD solution you will soon develop a feel for the color and so the chlorine dioxide gas content. You can use CDSplus with 0.29% chlorine dioxide solution as a color reference: with CDSplus it is pretty certain that the contents comprise what is stated on the label. In this way you can basically gain orientation for future reference. Otherwise, devices such as the "Dr. Nüsken photometer"

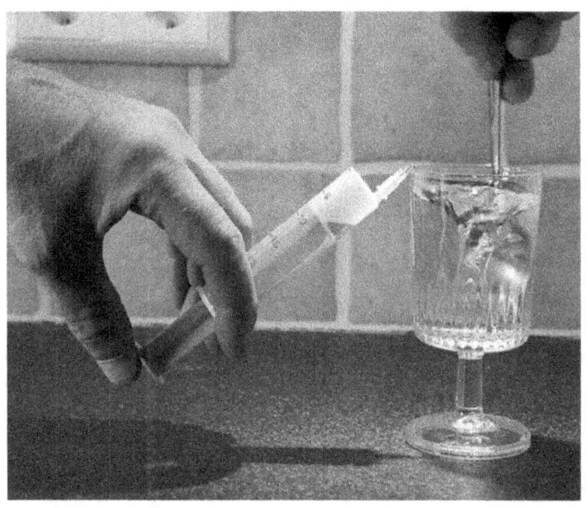

or for professional use the high-end "Palintest" are to be recommended for measuring the chlorine dioxide content.

Once this process is complete, remove the syringe, carefully extract the plunger, and dilute the contents in water, which can be then disposed of or used as a disinfectant.

I wish you success!

5.3 Preparing CDS in quantity oneself

In this chapter you will find instructions for preparing CDS in words and pictures. Needless to say, you can buy pre-prepared CDS or CDSplus. That is always the simplest way out. Preparing the solution oneself is most likely cheaper and ensures that it is fresh.

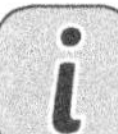

Preparation of CDS

Organize the following materials in advance:

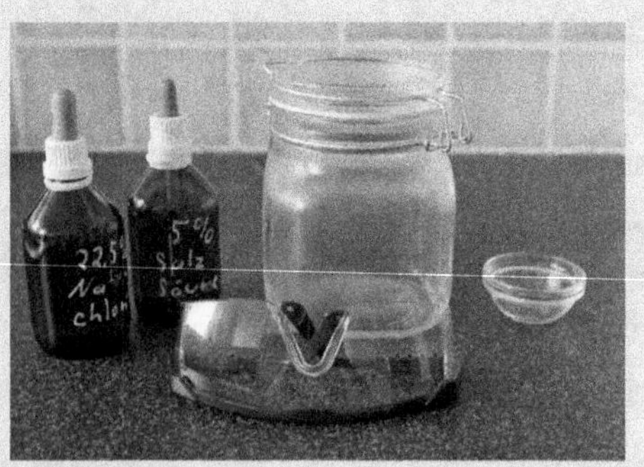

- Protective goggles
- Preserving jar with glass lid approx. 500 mL (16.907 fl oz)
- Glass bowl or similar - must not be perishable
- Sodium chlorite 22.5 %
- Acid, e.g., hydrochloric 5 - 10% or another acid (but not lactic acid for the production of gas is very slow)

1

Fill the preserving jar with water to just below the rim (you can see this clearly in the picture) and place the glass bowl inside. It is important that no water gets inside of the glass bowl!

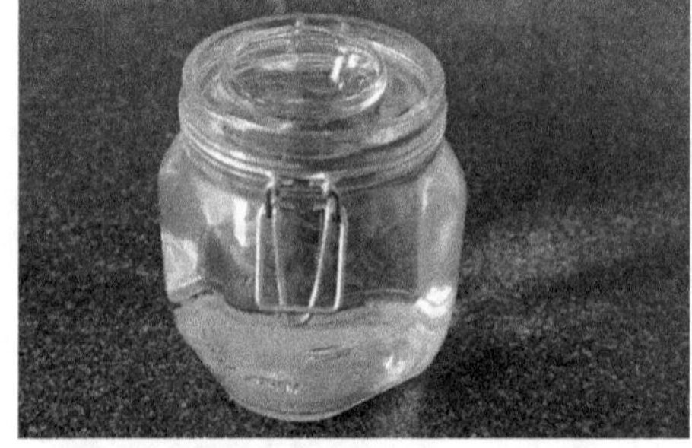

2

Put on the goggles to protect from any spray! This is essential as gas rises in the course of the activation process. Drip about five drops of sodium chlorite and five drops of hydrochloric acid into the glass bowl. The drops must come into contact with each other.

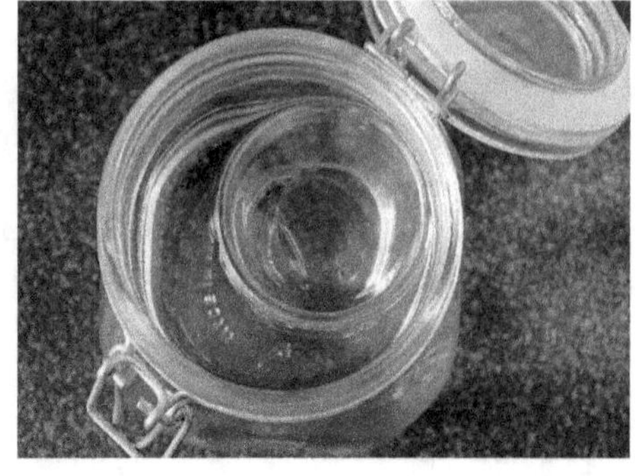

3

Close the lid and place the jar in the refrigerator. Take care that no water slops into the glass bowl!

The gas generated will now combine with the water.

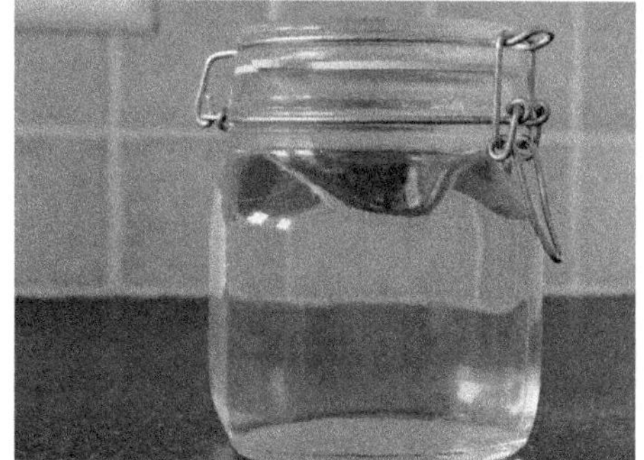

4

After around 30 minutes you will see that the water in the jar has turned yellow. The process is complete.

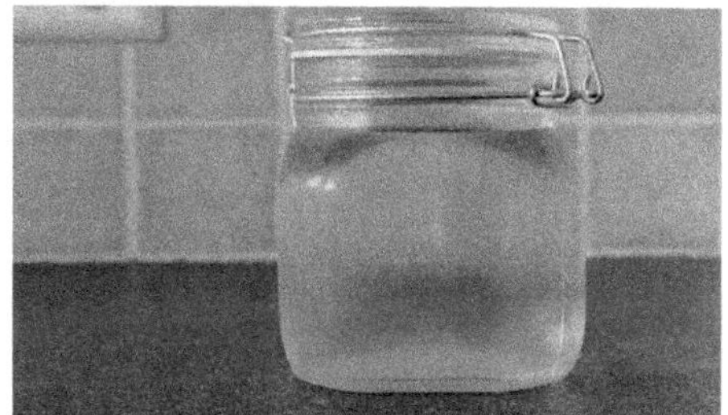

5

Leave the jar standing in the refrigerator overnight. Next day carefully remove the jar from the refrigerator. It remains important that neither the water sloshes into the bowl nor the fluid from the bowl splashes into the water. Put on the protective goggles again, open the lid, and carefully remove the bowl. The contents of the bowl must not run into the water. Take special care that no liquid makes contact with your skin! It is caustic! As for the contents of the glass bowl there are additional uses: Fill the bowl with water and put it in the refrigerator to kill germs or simply add it to your cleaning water. These are just two possibilities for use; there are many more.

The CDS produced can now be employed as usual.

Good Luck!

5.4 Preparing a chlorine dioxide infusion solution (CDI)[1]

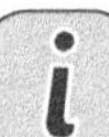

Materials for the preparation of a chlorine dioxide infusion solution

Material required for the preparation of an infusion:

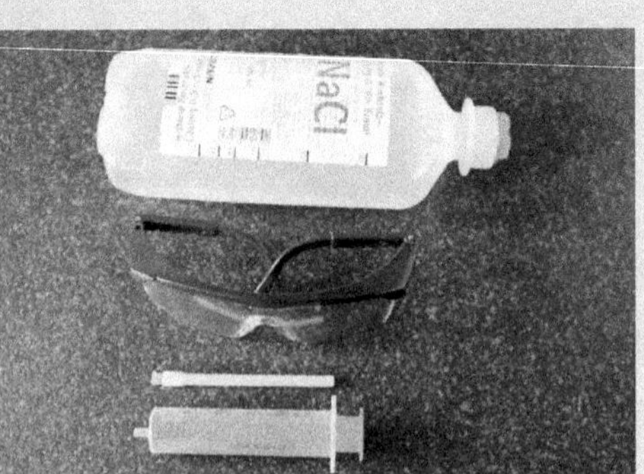

- Protective goggles
- Infusion solution
- Luer filter
- Syringe approx. 30 mL (1.014 fl oz)
- Hypodermic needle approx. 7 cm (2.75 in.)
- Sodium chlorite 22.5%,
- Acid, e.g., 5 - 10 % hydrochloric

acid or another acid (but not lactic acid as the production of gas is slow).

1

First put on the protective goggles and then press the needle with the Luer filter attachment onto the syringe. Draw the plunger out of the syringe and hold the opening facing up. Add five drops of sodium chlorite to the syringe and then five drops of acid, the sodium chlorite should not yet make contact with the acid. Press the plunger in a few millimeters more and gently rotate the syringe.

Now the sodium chlorite will mix with the acid to produce chlorine dioxide. Do not press the plunger in yet, wait for the gas to build (see "Preparing CDS in quantity oneself " Chapter 5.3).

---

1 CDI is the abbreviation for chlorine dioxide infusion solution. This is consists of a common cooking salt solution enriched with chlorine dioxide. One can quickly and efficiently go to the source of the malady this way.

Remove the sleeve from the needle and stick the needle into the infusion solution. One could insert a Luer filter between the syringe and needle to assure that no impurities sully the infusion solution.

2

Gently squeeze the gas into the infusion solution. Note! The reacting fluid must stay in the syringe!

Put the goggles on (you've most likely removed them). This process can if need be repeated to make a stronger solution. When finished, pull the syringe out of the infusion bottle. The chlorine dioxide infusion solution is prepared.

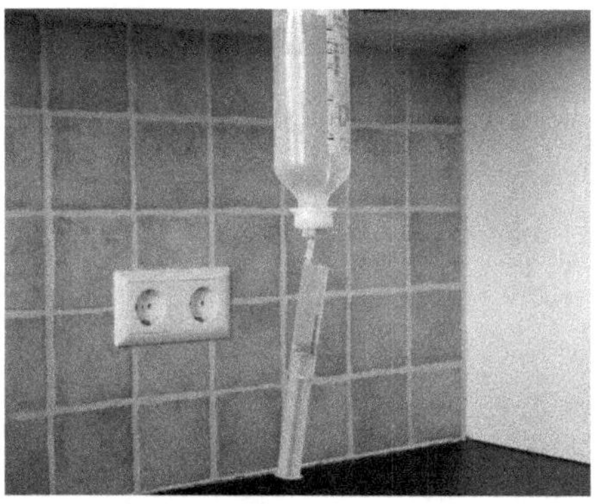
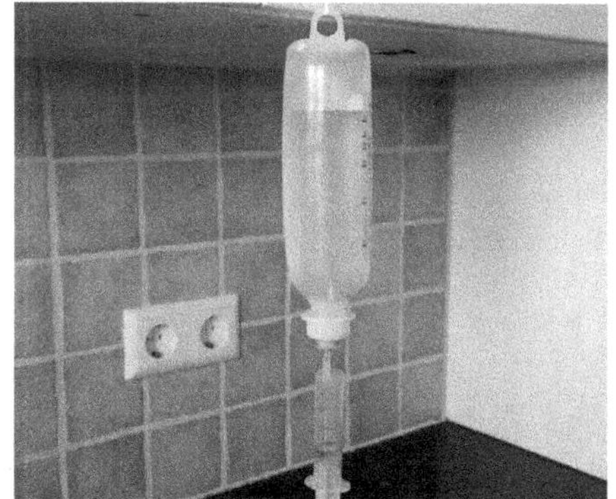

Add water to the syringe, throw the contents away or use it as disinfectant. To neutralize any possible chlorates add a drop of DMSO.[1]

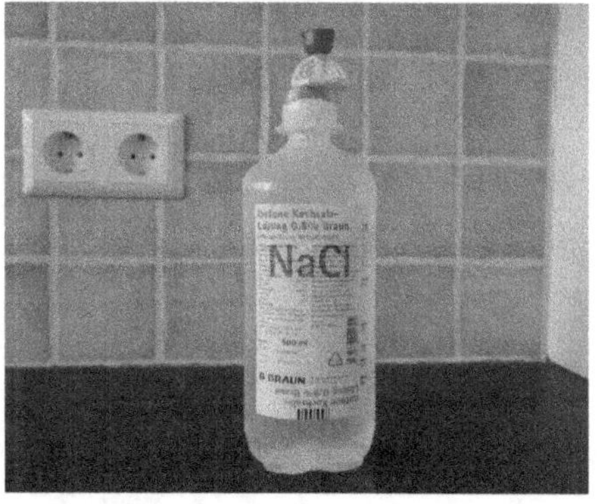

---

1 Cordial thanks to Wolfgang Stütz for his consent to use the images!

5.5 Preparing a Gefeu solution

Purchase a brown glass bottle at the drugstore, which has a volume of 100 to 110 mL (3.381 - 3.719 fl oz) and two disposal syringes of 10 mL (0.338 fl oz). The bottle should have a nozzle so that the Gefeu solution can later be measured out into a glass of water. This too can be purchased inexpensively at the drugstore.

Remove the nozzle from the bottle and put it aside, it will be set back in place following activation.

1

Measure out 20 mL (0.676 fl oz) cold water with the aid of a disposable syringe (10 mL/0.338 fl oz) and a fat needle (canula) from a glass of clean water and squirt the water into the glass bottle. Place the solution in the refrigerator! Put the bottles of sodium chlorite and acid in the refrigerator as well.

2

Take the second disposable syringe (10 mL/0.338 fl oz), and using a fat needle (canula) draw exactly 2 mL (0.067 fl oz) of MMS (22.5 % sodium chlorite solution) from the well-cooled bottle of sodium chlorite. To finish, carefully clean the needle with a paper towel.

3

Immediately after, stick the same needle into the similarly well-cooled bottle of acid and draw out precisely 2.4 mL (0.811 fl oz) of the 50% tartaric acid (or alternatively, hydrochloric acid 4 - 6%).

It is advisable to draw an extra 0.5 mL (0.017 fl oz) or so of air into the syringe thereby creating an air cushion to buffer the associated activation.

4

Now the sodium chlorite together with the 50% tartaric acid (or 3 - 4% hydrochloric acid) is activated in the syringe for exactly 30 seconds.

We can see the mixture in the syringe turn a yellow-red-brown color. This happens very quickly!
During the activation process droplets of the sodium chlorite being generated will leak from the needle as it turns gasiform.

5

We limit this by already inserting the needle into the almost horizontal brown bottle during activation in order that the chlorine dioxide released does not disperse into the air but is directed via the needle into the water and can bind there.

Please note! Take care that no water is able to dribble out of the bottle! A little creativity is called for! Hold the bottle firmly with one hand and the syringe with the other.

The largest possible amount of precious chlorine dioxide is won in this way.

6

After 30 seconds of activation squirt the total contents of syringe into the bottle with the pre-cooled water, replace the nozzle in the opening, replace the lid tightly, and shake the bottle a little. Put the bottle in the refrigerator right away!

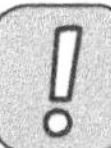

Clearly identify the bottle (e.g., write "Gefeu Solution" on an adhesive label) so that it will not be confused in the refrigerator with our bottle of MMS for instance!

As you see, it is not difficult to prepare a Gefeu solution. You can use all common acids such as 50% tartaric acid, or citric acid, or 4 6% hydrochloric acid for this purpose. Other recipes relating to the theme of "Gefeu" can be found at, for example, www.mmsselbsthilfe.de.

6
Practical Interaction with MMS

6.1 General interaction with MMS

The previous chapter contains all you need to know relating to the activation and application of MMS, CDS/CDSplus and Gefeu. Undoubtedly, you will have many questions such as: "How many drops can I give my horse and how often?" and "With which disorders can I use the medication?"

In this chapter I would like to demonstrate the practical uses of with MMS including several dosage recommendations. These are useful suggestions (rules of the thumb) as to dosage. A rule of thumb as to dosage is definitely always a great help, though the type and intensity of the illness as well as the particular animal are also significant as regards treatment. Should you work with the pendulum, the tensor, or with kinesiology, it is of advantage to test the dosage expressly for the animal. In doing so one can discern whether a cat, for instance, will tolerate a little or a lot on average. For those who are not in command of such capabilities I have put together a rough table as orientation. Trust your intuition and observe your animal. Consult a veterinarian or animal therapist if you feel uncertain.

Use these standardized guidelines. Better still test individually

What dose, and what should I bear in mind?

Animal	MMS	CDS	CDSplus	Gefeu
Small animal per 5 kg (11.023 lb)	1 drop	4 drops	4 drops	7 drops
Larger animal per 10 kg (22.046 lb)	1 drop	4 drops	4 drops	7 drops
Horse per 20 kg (44.092 lb)	1 drop	4 drops	4 drops	7 drops

It is simpler to dispense CDS and Gefeu: It is not necessary to activate; the number of drops can therefore be more easily regulated.

Important! Your animal's reactions and condition are the deciding factors, rather than these rules of thumb. Always pay heed to your animal. Before you begin you can read some more tips in Chapter 14 "Animal Communication."

I readily recommend CDS and CDSplus to my clients, as implementation is simpler. By administering CDS and CDSplus unpleasant reactions such as diarrhea and vomiting can be avoided.

6.1.1 Potential reactions

It goes without saying that it is a reasonable and normal expectation that the medicine helps in the event you have done everything correctly. A list of possible symptoms to watch out for follows:

Increase the dosage too much and too quickly and it may come to pass that the body is not done with the excretion; stomachache, vomiting or diarrhea may occur as a result.

> **Observe your animals attentively and decrease the dose in cases of queasiness, vomiting and/or diarrhea right away. Given even signs of a slight stomachache or gagging it is best to respond. Also note that horses and hares, for instance, cannot vomit. Exercise special care with these animals.**

What do I do when my animal suffers from severe diarrhea or vomiting?

It is important to observe the animal. Often things are not as bad as seems at first. It is a reaction. The body disposes too quickly and does not keep up with the evacuation. Whether the symptoms appear just one time or continue longer is vital. To follow is a guide to how to best respond in such a situation:

Optimal response to when severe diarrhea or vomiting occurs
Appropriate response on the basis of a dog weighing approx. 30 kg (66.138 lb):

Day	Dose	Amount of water	Times per day	Reaction
Day 1	4 drops CDS/CDSplus	50 ml (1.690 fl oz)	3 x	
Day 2	8 drops CDS/CDSplus	50 ml (1.690 fl oz)	3x	
Day 3	12 drops CDS/CDSplus	100 ml (3.381 fl oz)	3 x	Stool is mushy, though no diarrhea
Day 4	4–16 drops CDS/CDSplus	100 ml (3.381 fl oz)	3x	Stool is normal again, no diarrhea

If the stool on the third day has become thinner again, revert to eight drops and first increase gradually after two days. We watch our darling vigilantly.

Day	Dose	Amount of water	Times per day	Reaction
Day 5 - 6	8 drops CDS/CDSplus	50 ml (1.690 fl oz)	3 x	Stool is again normal
Day 7 -10	10 drops CDS/CDSplus	100 ml (3.381 fl oz)	3x	well accepted
Day 11 - 14	12 drops CDS/CDSplus	100 ml (3.381 fl oz)	3 x	general condition very good

What can I do when I have dispensed too much or the animal reacts with severe vomiting or retches?

In such cases case one can encourage the animal to drink water. With the aid of a disposable syringe squirt water directly into its mouth.

Bicarbonate of soda or vitamin C as antidote to over dosage!

Should an animal react with queasiness or vomiting to the smallest dose of MMS, CDSplus, CDS or Gefeu right away, then one can mix in bicarbonate of soda and make the solution less acid.

Mixing ratio (refer to "The MMS Handbook" by Dr. Antje Oswald, p. 105): 1 drop of MMS to 8 drops 10% bicarbonate of soda solution (1 level teaspoon of bicarbonate of soda to 9 teaspoons water).

With severe diarrhea or vomiting vitamin C can help. For humans 1 to 5 g (0.1690 fl oz) is recommended. It is better to increase the dose very gradually. Vomiting once only or suffering diarrhea for one day indicates a reaction. The medication is doing its job in our animal's body; the body cannot perform the "evacuation" of the refuse as quickly as required.

Another reaction can be blemished skin.

A considerable amount of detoxification is performed by the body's largest organ - the skin. This process can look like acne and/or engender itching. Don't panic! Even this is a positive reaction and will vanish once the detoxification process is complete. The treatment can be underpinned by washing with water fortified with MMS. These ablutions mitigate the symptoms and promote healing.

Often the animal owner seeks a rapid cure and therefore increases the dosage too quickly.

Detoxification takes time.

Even when your animal tolerates the increased dosage this will not result in faster recovery. It is likely that the animal will become listless and indolent, as the body cannot bring the inner process to end. If you notice that your animal is exhibiting such symptoms then please reduce the dosage! Too much can cause damage! The medicine is at work in the body and this process is strenuous for animals. The body must first come to terms with this before the powers of self-healing kick in. Please give yourself and your animal time. Be patient, even though this can be difficult at times.

What's wrong when it doesn't help?

The dose may be too high if it doesn't help.

Check whether or not the correct dosage is being administered. Maybe the dose is too low or too high.

Does MMS alone help with this illness?

Do I perhaps need additional medicines as back up? What can I change? Best consult a veterinarian or animal therapist who works with or is open to MMS; they can assist with the therapy and test for the appropriate accompanying medication.

Small miracles often come to pass rapidly, while the big ones take their own time.

6.1.2 Acids for activation

It is possible to activate sodium chlorite with various acids. Initially Jim Humble implemented vinegar. Then came 10% citric acid with a mixing ratio of 1:5. Most acids available today are called "1:1 activators." Conveniently, the same number of drops is dispensed from each bottle, i.e., 1 drop sodium chlorite and 1 drop acid. This applies to 50% citric acid and tartaric acid, 21% lactic acid, and 4 to 6% hydrochloric acid.

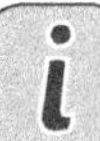

Lactic acid as a MMS activator - the activator of the future?

21% Dextrogyral (right-handed) lactic acid for the activation of sodium chlorite

Why lactic acid to activate?

Original quote from Dr. Hartmut Fischer (DMSO Handbook p. 102):
"As MMS is relatively often used by people who suffer from a malignant tumor I have come round to simply recommending the use of right-handed (dextrogyral) lactic acid as an activator.
Dextrogyral lactic acid can be administered therapeutically in its own right - one stone kills two birds in this way.

1. Lactic acid is an organic acid that reliably activates and simultaneously stabilizes MMS solution.
2. Lactic acid is a physiological substance that has diverse excellent signal detoxifying attributes regarding the human organism.
3. Lactic acid, being a prebiotic, supports enteric flora critical to the immune system."

Using any of these acids can activate sodium chlorite. Hydrochloric acid is among the best of the activators, delivering a quick, clean and taste-neutral reaction.

Many prefer dextrorotatory d-tartaric acid in that it is a natural product and reacts quickly, but it must not be left to activate for more than a minute for it will crystalize. Lactic acid reacts slowly, but long term (retard). Quick acids are called for when one wishes to release as much chlorine dioxide as possible. Slow acids are called for in order to achieve a soft, slow, and controlled, i.e., ongoing effect. Generally though, almost all acids work.

You can use right-handed (dextrogyral) lactic acid (RMS) 1:1 in the manner of the other already familiar activators.

Decide for yourself which the best option might be.

6.1.3 Overview of the acids table

Acid	Acid in %	Number of drops sodium chlorite	Number of drops acid	Mix ratio	Activation time
hydrochloric acid	4–6 %	1	1	1:1	30–45 sec
citric acid	50 %	1	1	1:1	30–45 sec
tartaric acid	50 %	1	1	1:1	30–45 sec
lactic acid	21 %	1	1	1:1	30–45 sec
citric acid	10 %	1	5	1:5	3 min
tartaric acid	10 %	1	5	1:5	1–3 min

Explanation: **What does the ratio designation indicate?**
Mix ratio "1:5" for example, indicates that one drop of sodium chlorite and five drops of activator are brought together.

6.1.4 Safety precautions

It is very important to keep medicines out of reach of children! CDSplus, CDS and Gefeu solution should be stored cool! With MMS (2 components) cool storage is not essential.

In that MMS and CDS possess very powerful active properties too much can be harmful. Due to their potency they are, among other purposes, employed in the fight against stubborn bacteria and viruses.

As in many other fields: Excess is equal to poison! Just as one "treat" per week is something special, the same each day can over an extended period harm the health of our animals.

Rules of thumb when using MMS

1. It is essential to calculate dosage according to body weight. Best begin with the smallest dose and increase gradually: Don't be unnecessarily ambitious!

2. Take care that neither chlorine dioxide nor sodium chlorite comes in contact with clothing! Both are corroding when undiluted and can cause discoloration.

3. Avoid breathing in fumes during activation. It is in fact helpful to puff out some breath across the opening of the glass following activation. Ideally, work next to an open window when activating MMS.

4. What to do when the dose was too high? Vitamin C, bicarbonate of soda, lots of water, zeolite, et cetera - all neutralize.

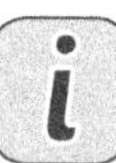

Continuation: Rules of thumb when using MMS

5. Note: The liquid derived from sodium chlorite and acid is caustic! This must first be diluted with water. With an increased number of drops the amount of water must also be increased. If I give a horse for instance 100 or more drops, it is not enough to dilute this with only 100 mL (3.381 fl oz) water - this may still be caustic.

   I witnessed this with a horse: The owner did not increase the amount of water enough and the horse's throat was burned a little. Caution is advised, but don't worry: This light burning healed within a few days.

6. Subsequent to the activation it is equally important not to breathe in the accrued chlorine dioxide that is now a gas. A longish inhalation of high concentration can be poisonous.

   (For more information see: "The MMS Handbook"
   by Dr. Antje Oswald, Daniel-Peter-Verlag)

6.1.5 Tips and tricks

In the following I would like to pass on a few tips and tricks that have occurred to me in the course of my work with animals. They have been of assistance to owners and to myself when treating animals.

a) Dispense MMS with a syringe

As a rule, I advise animal owners to administer MMS/CDS directly into the mouth with the aid of a syringe. This can with sensitive animals, especially cats, cause stress. Such stress can impede recovery or trigger new symptoms.

MMS/CDS dispensed directly into the mouth with the aid of a syringe

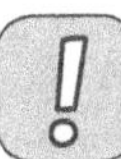

> In such cases it is better to mix MMS or CDS with some grainy cream cheese, cream thinned with water, or some other treat. This is then enthusiastically lapped up - the nerves of the animal and the animal owner are thus spared.

b) Treating the eyes of cats

Soak a cotton cloth in the solution

Treating the eyes of our cats we must be at times somewhat resourceful. Something that has proved to work well is to dip a small piece of cotton cloth (e.g., a diaper) in the pre-prepared solution and to press this gently onto the eyes; a little stroking of the tummy can be very helpful.

In that the such is generally not positively construed by stray cats one can effectively treat them by adding the medication to their food.

c) "Washing" cats

"Riot gear" is advisable

How do I wash a cat? Here, I must smile inwardly. I see myself in a chain-mail shirt, gauntlets, and other worthy articles of clothing out of medieval times. "Riot gear" might be of advantage here.

Squirt pre-prepared solution under the fur with a syringe without the needle

A better idea, I found out, is to squirt pre-prepared solution from a disposable syringe (without needle) under the fur, not on the skin, in small amounts. This is received well by cats when done with one hand while with the other simultaneously rubs in the lotion. By means of the ensuing grooming a little lotion enters the body as well.

d) Administering MMS to hares and guinea pigs

The administration of MMS/CDS to hares and guinea pigs can at times be problematic. As a rule the medicine is simply offered them by means of their drinking receptacle, but the smell can put them off from drinking. To overcome this, wet fodder (grass) can be withheld temporarily or completely and the intake of dry fodder (hay) accordingly increased; the animal is thus thirsty and will soon drink despite the odor.

Trick: Provide augmented dehydrated fodder…

e) Dosage and guidelines

Guidelines are principles whereby one can orient oneself. Not all animals will stomach the recommended dosage: One should start carefully and increase slowly - that is after all more acceptable to the animals.

Practice animal communication

The disparity between recommended dosages provided in reports is conspicuous, but every animal responds differently to MMS and other medicaments. I try to always adjust to the individual animal, customarily via animal communication (Chapter 14). During the initial exchange with the owner I often sense the animal is very sensitive. I do not begin with high doses in such cases, as the animal will react immediately by vomiting or with diarrhea. In that the animal is already weakened due to sickness it would be counterproductive for the treatment and a retrograde step in some cases. The dosage is first put to the test. At times the dosage might be, contrary to the guidelines, relatively high: my colleagues found that animals were responding well to these dosages.

Most importantly, one should always have in mind that the dosage prescribed helps and is not an uncalled-for burden.

f) Administering MMS with food

Augmentation by way of the food is sometimes necessary.

At the outset it is said that it is beneficial to dispense MMS separately to the feed, and yes, to do so is best and more effective.

Regrettably, it is often not all that simple in practice. Some animals due to prolonged treatment involving tablets and shots are already ill disposed and others simply avoid anything that does not taste like their customary food. In order to be able to administer it at all it is preferable to dispense MMS along with their food.

When in doubt, call on a therapist or veterinarian who uses MMS!

g) Administering to rabbits

Stroke the bunny with one hand and administer the syringe to its mouth

I can offer you a little ploy for administering MMS to rabbits; dexterity and a little practice are required.

Hold the rabbit on your lap, stroke its flank with one hand and with the other slowly press the solution out of the syringe into its mouth. A natural response is induced due to the stroking and the animal will start to lick.

h) Administering powders, such as anthelmintics (deworming medicine)

Natural yoghurt or sour cream as a lure

Very effective herbal anthelminthics (e.g. CdVet - WurmoVet) are available, plant-based mixes as well. One hint for cat owners is to mix these herbal or plant dewormers in with yoghurt or sour cream (or something similar). Cats can be outsmarted this way, mostly. One needs be inventive with cats, always come up with something new.

i) Administering amino acids, vitamins, et cetera.

The body is thoroughly cleansed by MMS. Due to being ill and the subsequent process of self-healing the body loses lots of amino acids, vitamins, and so forth. Hence it is important to resupply these to the body. In this connection assorted items such as moringa oleifera and fresh or dried herbs have proven themselves to be reliable. The palette is large and can thus be fine-tuned to the particular animal being treated.

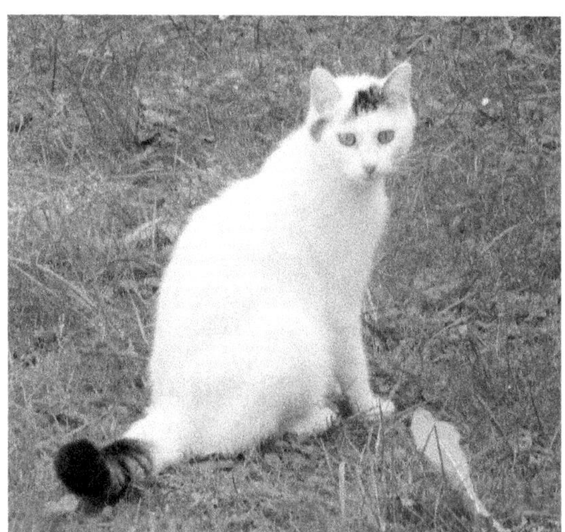

k) Dispensing CDS to cats

The implementation of chlorine dioxide can be difficult with cats. This was especially awkward on one occasion. This cat ate only dry food and would not accept treats such as cream (or the like) or liverwurst. You name it: Madame refused all that was not her familiar dried food. So we would place a couple of drops on her paws, which she then licked clean - recovery took a long while, but ultimately progress was good.

Put a couple of drops on the paws

6.2 Standard instructions (protocols) for humans

The protocol for humans of about 70 kg (154.323 lb) can be adapted to suit animals according to purpose and weight.

6.2.1 MMS protocol 1000 and application (for humans)

Recurrent saturation of the blood

The advantage of MMS Protocol 1000: It has been demonstrated that a small dose taken regularly occasions greater success than a single higher dose. There are many pathogens cocooned in the cells that first multiply and then stream forth. As chlorine dioxide does not attack cells it is effective only when the pathogens leave the cells. Hence, a recurrent saturating of the blood, especially when dealing with difficult to reach and persistent pathogens such as Lyme borrelia leads to focused eradication.

The Protocol 1000 is the standard protocol and is a guide to the intake of MMS, not mandatory. The dosage can be altered to suit the individual. It is however the appropriate protocol in many cases.

1 activated drop/hours per 8 hours/day over 3 days

- 2 activated drops/hours per 8 hours/day over 4 days

- 3 activated drops/hours per 8 hours/day over 7 days

Activting MMS

Put 1 - 3 drops of sodium chlorite and 1 - 3 drops of activator in a dry glass, and wait 30 - 45 seconds. Holding the glass at an angle, gently rotate it until the drops turn to an amber color. Top up with 150 - 200 mL (5.072 - 6.762 fl oz) cold water and drink immediately.

Daily supply

It is advisable to prepare a 1 Liter (33.814 fl oz) glass water bottle with a plastic lid containing say 24 drops of MMS for the whole day; this can then be marked with 7 stripes. It is then easy to drink the hourly dose at work, at the office, or in school without needing to activate each time. Besides, the taste, energy usage and palatability are better when the mixture is prepared the evening before and stored in the refrigerator until required. Another advantage is that one must not repeatedly activate; the mixture is however not as strong and fresh.

A 1 Liter (33.814 fl oz) glass water bottle: Provisions for work, the office and school

Recommendations

- Do not drink juices containing artificial vitamin C supplements for one hour before taking your medication.
- Drink plenty of still water - a minimum of 2 - 3 Liters daily, more will do no harm.
- Take MMS and anticoagulants at separate times. No interactions with other medications, homeopathic medicines included, have been observed. MMS thins the blood as well, and may thus increase the effects of anticoagulants. To avoid the blood becoming too thin, extra caution is advised.

MMS thins the blood.

Mixing ratio, activator and activation time

Hydrochloric acid is recommended as an activator as it is naturally present in the stomach and leaves no by-products. Lactic acid is preferable in relation to skin symptoms as well as cancer. Citric acid is not ideal as it is harsh. Citric acid produces by-products that can stress the body - this acid is namely not derived from lemons, but often cultured using mold fungus (Aspergillus niger).

Citric acid is not ideal.

- With 4% hydrochloric acid, 21% lactic acid, 50% tartaric acid, and 50 % citric acid:
  1:1 / 30 - 45 sec. activation time
- With 10% citric acid and lemon juice:
  1:5 / 3 minutes activation time

Prolongation

The 1000 protocol can be extended for three weeks or longer.

The protocol 1000 can be augmented to the extent that one either increases the number of drops per hour to 8 hours/day, or maintains the amount of drops and increases the dosage to 12 single doses/day, or applies both. Further, one can extend the 1000 protocol to three weeks or longer, though a break of one or two days at the end of two weeks does the body no harm. In addition, as a change, one can undertake a cure involving strong antioxidants.

6.2.2 CDS 101 protocol according to Dr. Andreas Kalcker (for humans)

The CDS 101 protocol is analog to the MMS 1000 protocol.

The CDS 101 protocol is the analog to the MMS 1000 protocol, the distinction being that CDS or CDSplus are utilized.

1. 10 mL (0.338 fl oz) CDS (2900 ppm i.e. 0.29 %), equivalent to approx. 200 drops in 1 Liter (33.814 fl oz) water. This is the daily ration.
2. Divide this into eight to twelve measures and drink a portion hourly.

Important: Always pay attention to the body!

The dose can be increased case-by-case and according to health: It is important to pay attention to the body. Should dizziness or fatigue occur revert immediately to the previously dosage tolerated.

6.2.3 Protocol MMS 1000 + (MMS + DMSO as adjuvant) for humans

For tenacious viruses such as herpes or funguses: Activate MMS drops with acid for 45 seconds. Add the desired amount of water and the same number of drops (as MMS) of DMSO. Stir well, and drink.

Treatment of stubborn viruses.

Step 1:	3 drops MMS
Step 2:	3 drops acid, e.g., 4% hydrochloric acid, 21% lactic acid, or 50% citric acid or tartaric acid
Step 3:	activation 45 seconds
Step 4:	add 100 mL (3.381 fl oz) water
Step 5:	3 drops DMSO in the mixture
Step 6:	stir well and drink

An example:

DMSO functions here as a transporter, or as I like to say: "door opener." It enables MMS to enter the tissue more rapidly and deeper and to find its way to the "hot-spot." A further advantage is that DMSO has anti-inflammatory and analgesic properties.

DMSO as "door opener"

6.3 Standard instructions for animals

To follow are some rules of thumb with respect to dosage. For additional information see: Chapter 6.1.

Dosage: Rules of for oral administration

Small animals	1 drop MMS (4 drops CDS, 4 drops CDSplus, 7 drops Gefeu) per 5 kg (11.023 lb) plus 10 mL (0.338 fl oz) water
Larger animals	1 drop MMS (4 drops CDS, 4 drops CDSplus, 7 drops Gefeu) per 10 kg (22.046 lb) plus 10 mL (0.338 fl oz) water
Horses	1 drop MMS (4 drops CDS, 4 drops CDSplus, 7 drops Gefeu) per 20 kg (44.092 lb) plus10 mL (0.338 fl oz) water

6.3.1 Eye and ear drops, and spray general

You will need: 1 drop MMS (activated), or 4 drops CDS/CDSplus and 10 mL (0.338 fl oz) water

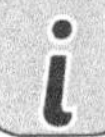

Preparing eye drops

You need a small, brown 50 mL (1.690 fl oz) glass bottle with spray attachment or dropper (available at drugstores).

1. Activate 1 drop MMS with the activator, or use 4 drops CDS. With CDS omit point 3.

2. Wait for the activation of MMS and the acid to happen (Chapter 7.1.2).

3. To conclude, add 10 mL (0.338 fl oz) water to the activated drops. Fasten the attachment and commence treatment.

6.3.2 Eye and eardrops with DMSO

For purulent eye or ear inflammation and mites in the ear, MMS drops with added DMSO have been shown to be effective.

1 drop MMS (activated)	or 4 drops CDS/CDSplus
1 drop DMSO	1 drop DMSO
10 mL water (0.338 fl oz)	10 mL water (0.338 fl oz)

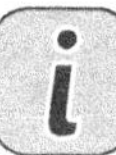

Preparing eye drops with DMSO

You will need a small, 50 mL (1.690 fl oz) brown glass bottle and a glass pipette (available from drugstores).

1. In the 50 mL (1.691 fl oz) bottle activate 1 drop MMS with acid (Chapter 6.1.2), or use 4 drops of CDS or CDSplus.

2. Add 10 mL (0.338 fl oz) water.

3. Add 1 drop of DMSO to the solution.

4. Finally, employing the pipette drip the solution drop by drop into the eye (or the ear).

With cats especially, treating the eyes is tricky. Here it is usually preferable to take a scrap of cotton fabric (e.g., a piece of baby diaper), dip it in the solution, and gently press it onto the eye; a little tummy-rub will be of assistance. Even a light wiping with the cloth can bring very good results. Spraying can help with strays.

6.3.3 Wound spray general

5 drops MMS (activated)	or 20 drops (2 mL/0.067 fl oz) CDS
½ mL (0.017 fl oz) DMSO (approx. 10 drops)	½ mL (0.017 fl oz) DMSO(approx. 10 drops)
100 mL water (3.381 fl oz)	100 mL water (3.381 fl oz)

This mixture can be kept at ready in a glass spray-bottle and sprayed several times a day. It is often helpful to carefully dab small wounds with a scrap of cotton fabric, e.g., a diaper.

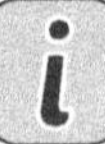

Preparing a wound spray

You will need a glass spray-bottle of approx. 500 mL (16.907 fl oz)

1. Activate 5 drops of MMS with acid (See: Chapter 6.1.2) or 20 drops of CDS/CDSplus.

2. After activation (Chapter 6.1.2) add 100 mL (3.381 fl oz) water.

3. Now add 10 drops (½ mL/0.017 fl oz) of DMSO. Attach the spray-head and tend to the wound.

6.3.4 Washes general

20 drops MMS (activated)	or 80 drops (4 mL /0.135 fl oz) CDS or CDSplus
5 L water (1.320 gal)	5 L water (1.320 gal)

> **Preparing a solution for washes**
>
> You will need a 10 L (2.641 gal) bucket.
>
> 1. Activate 20 drops of MMS with acid (See: Chapter 6.1.2), or use 4 mL (0.135 fl oz) of CDS/CDSplus.
>
> 2. Following activation (Chapter 6.1.2), add 5 Liter (1.320 gal) water. You can effectively wash dogs and horses suffering from skin disorders using a cotton towel or wash-mitt. With cats, which famously will not be bathed under any circumstances, or only when the owner is clad in "riot gear," it has been shown that a little solution sprayed from a disposable syringe (without needle!) in small amounts, under the fur and not onto the skin, while simultaneously rubbing in the solution, can work. In course of the ensuing grooming a certain amount of the MMS or CDS solution will enter the body.

6.3.5 Tabular overview: Standard recommendations for animals for external application

	MMS	or CDS /CDSplus	+ DMSO	Water
Eyes / ears, Drops without DMSO	1 drop	4 drops		10 mL (0.338 fl oz)
Eyes / ears Drops with DMSO	1 drop	4 drops	1 drop	10 mL (0.338 fl oz)
Wound spray	5 drops	20 drops/1 mL (0.033 fl oz)	1½ mL (0.050 fl oz) DMSO (approx. 10 drops)	100 mL (3.381 fl oz)
Wash	20 drops/1 mL (0.034 fl oz)	80 drops/4 mL (0.135 fl oz)		5 L (1.320 gal)

6.3.6 CDS injections according to Dr. Andreas Kalcker

This is a protocol for mammals. For 80 kg (176.369 lb) live-weight between 2 - 5 mL (0.067 - 0.169 fl oz / 40 to 100 drops) CDI (chlorine dioxide injection) 3000 ppm (0.29% chlorine di-

Intramuscular and intravenous application

oxide solution) 1:5, is diluted with 10 - 25 mL (0.338 - 0.845 fl oz) table salt solution and administered intravenously or intramuscularly. Please always match the dose to the current weight of the animal. As an alternative, one can inject up to a maximum of 15 mL (0.507 fl oz) into a 1 Liter (33.814 fl oz) bag of common table salt and use this as an infusion. This can be used as a daily ration. Pains in the veins may come about with prolonged use, therefore the pH value should always be tested: pH 7 is optimal. In the case of low pH values add 1 to 3 drops of sodium chlorite ($NaCIO_2$) to slowly increase the value to pH value 7. The solution is in itself sterile due to the chlorine dioxide, and to eliminate the pyrogens employ a Luer filter as a syringe add-on (between syringe and needle; available at drugstores). For detailed instructions for preparation of CDI solution see p. 110.

6.4 Standard instructions general, by animal

To follow are protocols that enable the commencement of treatment. Each protocol should certainly be considered and then field-tested, the particular animal is of primary importance: How is it and how does it react? What is good for one animal is not the same for another. For that reason it is most important to observe the animal and trust your intuition. In the case studies the findings are very divergent.

Most important is the animal itself.

6.4.1 Standard instructions dogs

| Small dog | begin with 1 drop MMS | or with 4 drops CDS/CDSplus |
| Big dog | begin with 2 drop MMS | or with 8 drops CDS/CDSplus |

It is best to activate the MMS in a small shot glass, half fill this with water, suck this into a 10 mL (0.338 fl oz) disposable syringe (without needle), and then dispense this directly into the dog's mouth. Do this three times a day at first, then increase the dose by one drop daily to reach the targeted amount. With small dogs increase the dose carefully - increasing the amount every 2 or 3 days is often more agreeable. With small dogs dispensing CDS/CDSplus is better suited and simpler to dose. An hourly dose, circa six times per day has been proven to bring very positive results in acute cases; cancer, leishmaniasis, or the like. This dose can be maintained for one or two days, followed by three times daily for up to two weeks.

Activate in a shot glass

As always it is very important to note: This is but ONE option as regards dosage, the individual animal must be taken into account. Be it nausea, vomiting, gagging or diarrhea please respond immediately and reduce the dose! Keep in mind: Less is often more!

Calculate the maximum dosage according to bodyweight. The rule of thumb is 1 activated drop of MMS or 4 drops of CDS/CDSplus to 10 kg (22.046 lb) bodyweight. Maintain this dosage for one to two weeks - here too, "can" is the operative word! Please take special care as regards horses and other animals that do not vomit to set the limit low; we have determined that often a few drops suffice to restore health. Some animals do not tolerate the suggested dose, or the dosage should be increased gradually and very carefully. I repeat: Important! Be watchful and if necessary please consult a therapist with knowledge of these substances, your animal will thank you.

6.4.2 Standard instructions Cats

Cats	4 drops CDS/CDSplus	3 x daily

In acute cases one can try to dispense the dose more often. Here is another rule of thumb: 20 drops CDS = 1 mL (0.033 fl oz)

For cats, I mostly recommend administering CDS/CDSplus as it is simpler to measure out and cats find it more agreeable. Should your cat react badly to 4 drops, it is a breeze to reduce the dose to 2 drops. The maximum dose is calculated according to bodyweight as well (max. 3 drops MMS or 12 drops CDS/CDSplus). Observe your cat. Neither you, nor a protocol determines the dose, but the cat alone. How is it? How does it respond to the medicine?

As mentioned above: Administering with a syringe, for cats, is frequently associated with great stress, which can show up negatively as concerns its overall condition. Here I find that with a small dish of CDS/CDSplus, some water and a little cottage cheese or the like, it all goes much more easily. Mostly, they lap it up eagerly. This is a proven method of treatment with wildcats as well.

As preventive treatment, cats and dogs can be given filled in their drinking bowl: 2 drops MMS (activated), or 8 drops CDS in a Liter (33.814 fl oz) of water. Adjust for smaller quantities accordingly.

6.4.3 Standard instructions horses

Phase	MMS activated	or CDS/CDSplus
Initially: mornings and evenings	10 drops in 200 mL (6.763 fl oz) water	40 drops in 200 mL (6.763 fl oz) water
Increase per day	+ 10 drops + 100 mL (3.381 fl oz) water	+ 40 drops (2 mL/0.067 fl oz) + 100 mL (3.381 fl oz) water
Maximum dose	50 drops + 600 mL (20.288 fl oz) water	200 drops (10 mL/0.338 fl oz) + 600 mL (20.288 fl oz) water

Begin with 10 drops of MMS activated with acid, or 40 drops (2 mL/0.067 fl oz) CDS/CDSplus, and 200 mL (6.763 fl oz) of water, morning and evening.

Increase daily by 10 drops of activated MMS or 40 drops (2 mL/ 0.067 fl oz) CDS. Frequently, an increase of up to 50 drops of activated MMS (maximum dosage) or 200 drops / 10 mL (0.338 fl oz) CDS/ CDSplus, administered for one to two weeks twice each day, is sufficient.

Day 1: 10 drops activated MMS or 40 drops (2 mL/0.067 fl oz) CDS/CDSplus + 200 mL (6.763 fl oz) water or apple juice (without vitamin C supplement).

Day 2: 20 drops activated MMS or 80 drops (4 mL/0.135 fl oz) CDS/CDSplus + 300 mL (10.144 fl oz) water or apple

juice (without vitamin C supplement).
Increase MMS and water until the maximum dose
is reached.

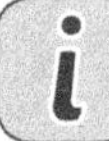

Tips for horses

The administration of MMS together with wheat bran is readily accepted. With the aid of a syringe (without needle) the mix can be directed into the mouth also; extra large horse syringes are available. The maximum dosage is very dependent on the individual, its weight and ailment. Most important with horses is careful consideration and under some circumstances a gradual build up for our lovely horses are unable to vomit.

6.4.4 Standard instructions hares, rabbits, guinea pigs, parrots ...

Hare/rabbit Guinea pig Parrot	4 drops CDS/CDSplus in ½ L water (16.907 fl oz)	distribute through the day

With small animals such as hares, rabbits, guinea pigs and parrots administer four drops of CDS/CDSplus in a half Liter of water that can then be readily filled in the drink receptacle. In many cases this will suffice as the maximum dose.

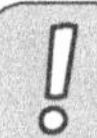

Should the animal refuse the water due to the smell, hares, rabbits or guinea pigs can be fed more dry food like such as hay while leaving grass out. The animal is thus thirstier and will drink despite the smell. Here too an incremental approach is vital.

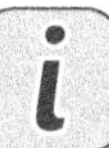

Replenishing the reserves of nutrients

In addition, it is important to bear in mind that the body due to "purification" with MMS, illness, and the process of self-healing too, loses large amounts of amino acids, vitamins and so forth. The body needs to be restocked. Products derived from Moringa Oleifera, for instance, and fresh or dried herbs, are most beneficial.

6.4.5 Standard instructions: Bees

This standard guide derives from the book by Dr. Antje Oswald: "The MMS Handbook," p. 196.

Bees	per 10 kg (22.046 lb) bee fodder	18 drops activated MMS, or 72 drops CDS/CDSplus

Word regarding the attributes of CDS, CDSplus and MMS has gotten round among beekeepers as well: Several beekeepers are investigating the use of MMS with their bees. First findings are expected in 2016.

6.4.6 Standard instructions pigeons

Phase	MMS activated	or CDS/CDSplus
to start: morning and evening	2 drops in 4 L (135.256 fl oz) water	8 drops in 4 L (135.256 fl oz) water
maximum dosage	6 drops in 4 L (135.256 fl oz) water	24 drops in 4 L (135.256 fl oz) water

When treating pigeons it is wise to begin with caution and accustom them slowly. Antje Oswald writes in her book "The MMS Handbook" that accustomization takes somewhat longer. Dosage: 6 drops of MMS or 24 drops CDS/CDSplus to 4 Liter (135.256 fl oz) water; filled in their drinking receptacle.

Pigeons slowly become accustomed to the medium dosage

This is the maximum dose; start with 2 drops of MMS or 8 drops of CDS/CDSplus and increase slowly.

6.4.7 Standard instructions tick bites general

MMS	CDS/CDSplus	Water	Dosage
6 drops	24 drops	200 mL (6.673 fl oz)	3

Ticks do not like MMS or DMSO.

Ticks happily bite horses, dogs and cats - often small "bumps" are left behind. These spots frequently itch, become inflamed due to being licked and bitten, and at times develop into an open wound. I recommend, even in the run-up, preparing a glass of water with 6 drops of MMS or 24 drops of CDS/CDSplus and that this be dabbed onto the area several times a day (cover the glass between treatments to prevent the gases escaping). I have noticed that animals with a healthy metabolism and immune system attract few or no ticks. There is also no cause to fear bites, only in the rarest case will Lyme disease (borreliosis) manifest. Most bites are relatively harmless, and cause only itching and some mild reddening. Here I would like to advise you of a commendable book: "Heal Borreliosis Naturally" (Borreliose natürlich heilen) by Wolf-Dieter Storl (See: Bibliography). One positive effect that I can attest to is that when DMSO and MMS are in use few or no tick bites appear.

6.4.8 Standard guide: Wounds general

DMSO as a natural analgesic and anti-inflammatory for wounds

According to the size of the wound a solution of MMS or CDS/CDSplus and water is mixed and the wound washed out. DMSO mixed in is a very helpful adjunct. The wound will be thus disinfected, any germs and bacteria will be eliminated, and the wound can heal faster. A few drops can be orally administered in addition. This must be adjusted according to the size and weight of the animal. Should the wound demand veterinary care, then begin with MMS afterwards - healing is encouraged and further treatment with antibiotics forestalled and/or the already administered medication cleared out. Antibiotics enfeeble the immune system and the body unlearns how to activate its self-healing processes.

MMS	or CDS/CDSplus	+ DMSO	+ Water
10 drops	40 drops 2 mL (0.067 fl oz)	20 drops 1 mL (0.033 fl oz)	200 mL (6.673 fl oz)

6.4.9 Tabular overview: Standard guide for animals internal usage

Animal	Weight	dosage MMS or CDS/CDSplus				Water	Times	Period
		to begin		maximum				
		MMS	CDS	MMS	CDS			
Small dog	approx. 10 kg (22.046 lb)	1 drop	4 drops	2 drops	8 drops	10 mL (0.338 fl oz)	3 x daily	1–2 weeks
Big dog	approx. 50 kg (110.231 lb)	1 drop	8 drops	5 drops	20 drops	10 - 100 mL (0.338 - 3.381 fl oz)	3 x daily	1–2 weeks
Cats	approx. 4 kg (8.818 lb)	½ drop	2 drops	2 drops	8 drops	10 mL (0.338 fl oz)	3 x daily	1–2 weeks
Horses	approx. 500 kg (1102.312 lb)	10 drops	40 drops (2 mL/ 0.068 fl oz)	250 drops	50 ml (1.6907 fl oz)	200 - 500 mL (6.763 - 16.907 fl oz)	2 x daily	1–2 weeks
Hares/ Rabbits	2 kg (4.409 lb)	1 drop	4 drops	1 drop	4 drops	500 mL (16.907 fl oz)	in drinking container	1 week
Parrots	not relevant	1 drop	4 drops	1 drop	4 drops	500 mL (16.907 fl oz)	in drinking container	1 week
Bees	not relevant	18 drops	72 drops	18 drops	72 drops	10 kg (22.046 lb) bee feed	in drink receptacle	feeding time
Pigeons	not relevant	2 drops	8 drops	6 drops	24 drops	4 L (135.256 fl oz)	in drinking container	always available

7 Large Practical Section: Applications

Introduction

The examples presented in the following derive from my practice and from colleagues, private persons and the veterinarian Dr. Schrader. Often my colleagues do not adhere to the standard protocols in that other agents like Bach flower extracts, plant tinctures and homeopathy are utilized, as well as animal communication. Furthermore, the dosage is at times adjusted to suit the specific animal. Myself, I view each animal individually and then decide how the therapy should proceed and be imparted to the owner.

Chapter 7 is based on experiences from my own practice and that of colleagues, private persons and the veterinarian Dr. Schrader.

The owner must not be disregarded as concerns the dosage of MMS, CDS, CDSplus or DMSO. Based on the accounts, you will certainly appreciate that now and then the dosage is far too low! Although, when an owner is very nervous I sometimes begin with a small dose thus avoiding a first reaction, thereby enabling the owner's faith in the medication to develop - likewise with the therapy. It is evident to me that mostly, despite the small amount of MMS, CDS, CDSplus or DMSO, an improvement can already be discerned within a few days.

Trust is important: The owner's faith in the treatment has direct impact on the animal's behavior.

Should you be new to MMS, please keep to the protocol to begin. If uncertain, or you do not believe things are as they should be please contact a therapist, a natural health professional or a veterinarian who has experience with these medicines. A number of addresses are listed in Chapter 18. What's more, it is most important that you yourself decide for this medicine and take responsibility.

A good place to start: Keep to the protocol to begin.

You will find abundant information relating to MMS and dosage in the books: "MMS - Breakthrough" by Jim Humble; "CDS/

MMS: Health is Possible" (CDS/MMS: Heilung ist möglich) by Dr. Andreas Kalcker; "The MMS Handbook: Health as Personal Responsibility" (Das MMS: Handbuch: Gesundheit in eigener Verantwortung) by Dr. Antje Oswald; and The DMSO Handbook: Hidden Medical Knowledge from Nature (Das DMSO: Handbuch: Verborgenes Heilwissen aus der Natur) by Dr. Hartmut Fischer.

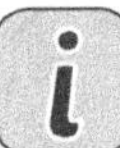

Rule of thumb for the mixing ratios of MMS, CDS/CDSplus and MMS 1

A simple rule of thumb is: For 10 kg (22.046 lb) weight employ 2 drops of MMS.
CDS/CDSplus is then 8 drops.
1 drop of MMS 1 is equivalent to 4 drops of CDS/CDSplus.

This is a rule of thumb only and must be adapted to each animal, its weight and the ailment. Generally CDS/CDSplus should be administered in even higher doses than four times the amount of MMS.

7.1 Dog illnesses that are successfully treated with MMS

7.1.1 Abscess following castration

Description practical example:

I treated a dog suffering from a dreadful abscess following castration. This burst and pus ran out resulting in two holes that I rinsed with activated MMS diluted in water. After three days it was healed. (See: "Standard instructions wounds general" Chapter 6.4.8).

7.1.2 Allergies

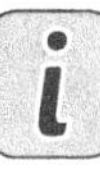

Allergy

Allergy (Greek: "allergos") meaning: "Different," "abundant," "overflowing."

To what does the allergy sufferer react to so "abundantly"?

Phenotype: Attacks of sneezing, itching, rash, diarrhea.
Causes: Continual overstimulation, poor diet, environmental pollution, many antibiotic regimes, pollution due to heavy metals.

What is an allergy?
An allergy is an overreaction by the immune system to normally harmLess substances. The origins are often poor nutrition, a weakened immune system due to vaccinations, pollution, emotional problems, et cetera.

Description practical example:

A dog diagnosed with grass allergy was brought to me. He had severe skin problems and suffered from intense itching. With the first visit I was looking at a fear ridden dog, one that to we humans might appear hugely amusing, especially when it is a massive Great Dane attempting to sit in mummy's lap. The root of the "allergy" was self-evident.

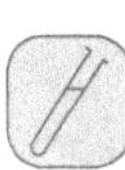

Treatment

First, I gave the dog a plant-based tincture, angelica tincture in this case, to boost its self-confidence.
Its skin condition was treated with a CDS wash, a mixture consisting of 20 drops of CDS in approximately 5 Liter (169.070 fl oz) water.
Seeing that this was a Great Dane the washing was easy to do, and already after a week the skin was healing. In addition, it was given Terrakraft extract to stimulate the metabolism. A couple of weeks later the fur was growing back.

7.1.3 Anus, inflamed

Description practical example:

As my dog aged he could no longer clean his anus properly, he accordingly became inflamed over and again. It was clear to me that he would be prescribed an antibiotic by the veterinarian and I wanted to avoid this. To spare the dog further inflammation I was obliged to squeeze the anal gland out. The final inflammation was treated in this way:

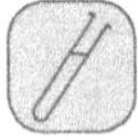

Treatment

I activated 4 drops of MMS with 4 drops of activator and diluted this with 10 mL (0.338 fl oz) water. I then dabbed the region with the solution.

The inflammation disappeared within a few days and no other problems materialized. Most important to me was the fact that no antibiotics were administered.

7.1.4 Anaplasmosis

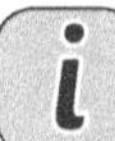

Anaplasmosis

The anaplasmosis, also called canine granulocytic ehrlichiosis, is caused by the bacteria of the family rickettsiaceae that is transferred by the tick type ixodes ricinus (castor bean tick). The transference takes place by means of the tick's saliva within a short period, 40 to 48 hours, subsequent to the bite. Ixodes ricinus is active when temperatures rise above 7 ºC (44 ºF), between March and November as a rule. The anaplasmosis attacks specific defense cells in the dog (neutrophils and eosinophilic granulocytes) and is borne by the blood to the various organs.

Description practical example:

A dog, approximately four years of age, and weighing about 12 kg (26.455 lb), diagnosed as having anaplasmosis. He had high temperature and was listless. In that this illness was bacterial it was treated as follows:

Treatment

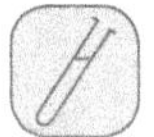

Day 1 + 2:   2 drops activated MMS mixed with approx. 10 mL (0.338 fl oz) water, administered directly into the mouth.

Day 3:   3 drops activated MMS mixed with 50 mL (1.69 fl oz) water, x 3 times.

Day 4:   4 drops activated MMS mixed with 50 mL (1.69 fl oz) water, x 3 times.

In addition, a teaspoon of zeolite in a little water was mixed in with the evening meal (approx. 1 hour after the final dose of MMS).

Even after a few days there were visible improvements. He was more agile and his temperature was in the region of normal; he found joy in life again. And now six months later, the dog exhibits no symptoms.

7.1.5 Respiratory tract infection according to veterinarian Dr. Schrader

Respiratory tract infection

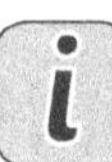

"With infections of the respiratory tract or the intestines bring 1 - 2 drops of 22.5% sodium chlorite solution into contact with 1 - 2 drops of 3.5% hydrochloric acid solution for exactly 1 minute (preferably use a common shot glass). By means of a syringe add approximately 2 - 5 mL (0.067 - 0.169 fl oz) tap water, disperse, draw the mix up into the syringe and administer the mixture directly into the mouth of the animal (at best sideways into the cheek pouch). This treatment should be undertaken after feeding (never on an empty stomach!). In extreme cases administer twice daily. Here too, harm to the patient was not evident at any time."

7.1.6 Eye infection

Description practical example:

The patient was a young Leonberger bitch with an ever-recurring eye infection. In addition, she was very unsure. She received daisies and angelica tincture for her psyche and Swedish bitters for her metabolism. After a week she was well and the eye infection was not apparent. The infection did not reappear.

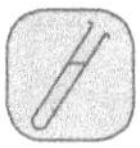

Treatment

We treated the eyes with homeopathic medicine: 16 drops of CDS mixed in a glass of water was dabbed on the eyes many times each day.

7.1.7 Bladder infection

Description practical example:

My dog was very unwell. I frequently came upon dribbles of urine. What's more, there was blood in the urine. Its temperature was high.

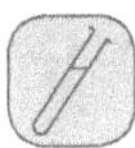

Treatment

I treated it immediately with CDS. Every 2 hours or so it was fed 4 drops of CDS mixed with a little water directly in the mouth. It is a miniature dachshund. The next day everything was already good. Just to be certain I gave it this dosage in the mornings and evenings for one week longer.

7.1.8 Lyme disease (Borreliosis)

Borreliosis

Borreliosis is conveyed through tick bites.

Phenotype: Fever, signs of paralysis, swollen lymph nodes.
Cause: Bacteria (borrelia) are conveyed via the bite; more precisely,
the tick attaching itself.

Description practical example:

One day I received a call from a distraught woman from Austria. *Case study:*
In tears, she told me that her dog, 2½ years old and weighing 35 *Paralyzed hips*
kg (77.162 lb), was paralyzed from the hips down. The veterinarian's diagnosis was an old and a new Borreliosis Titer as well as
an acute HD (hip dysplasia).

There was, according to the veterinarian, slim chance of recovery, and if there was no improvement he would accordingly put
the dog to sleep. Two days later I drove to Austria to look at the
problem. Via animal communication I found no indication of a
dysplasia. Following the initial conversation and clarification
of the diagnosis, I dispensed 2 drops of MMS, thinned it with
water and by means of a syringe (of course without the needle)
administered the mix straight into the dog's mouth on the spot.
After a short while he vomited profusely. The reaction of the
owner was: "Great, the garbage is coming out." When I told her
that her dog intended to walk on his own four legs to the next
visit to the veterinarian, I had learned this by means of the animal communication, she was very skeptical and would not believe me. I then discussed subsequent treatment with the owner.

I reduced the dosage due to the violent first reaction (see above):
A slow increase to 6 drops of MMS 3 times daily. Two days later
the dog owner rang: The dog after only one day of treatment

with MMS was able to stand unaided and after a week it could go outside alone to urinate and defecate.

The next visit to the veterinarian the dog walked on his own four legs, being put to sleep was no longer a consideration. The veterinarian's comment: "Well, the HD was not all that bad!?" No further comment.

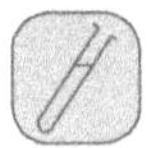

Treatment

Therapy plan:
Day 1: 3 x 2 drops MMS + activator + 30 mL (1.014 fl oz) water
Day 2: 3 x 4 drops MMS + activator + 30 mL (1.014 fl oz) water
Day 3: 3 x 6 drops MMS + activator + 30 mL (1.014 fl oz) water

This dose of 3 x 6 drops of activated MMS should be dispensed for two weeks. In this instance we activated the MMS with citric acid and diluted this with approximately 30 mL (1.014 fl oz) water. The solution was sucked up into a disposable syringe (without needle) and then slowly squirted directly into the animal's mouth.

Note: Clearly, the dosage was comparatively high. The dog tolerated the dosage very well, though this is too much for many dogs of similar weight. Please always observe the individual dog minutely.

7.1.9 Borreliosis with Alsatians

Excerpt from a client's letter:
"I believe I owe it to you and many others to communicate that by following your directions it has been possible to cure my German Shepherd (approximately 32 kg/70.547 lb) of borreliosis."

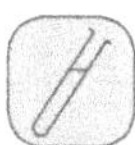

"I gave my dog 3 drops of MMS up to 9 times a day over 27 to 29 days.
He vomited only once following the sixth dose on the second or third day. I left him in peace for the rest of the day and gave him no more that day. On the aforementioned 27th or 28th day he suddenly refused the MMS and ran away from me. At this point his previously black belly had returned to being almost totally rosy, the symptoms had disappeared several days before. It was due only to my uncertainty and my being aware that borrelia can survive in the body, more specifically the joints, that I fed him MMS for so long."

"There has been no relapse or sign of borreliosis with my dog since July last year. He has put on weight and moves quite normally, plays ball, and enjoys his dog's life."

7.1.10 Chronic ear infection

See: "Ear infection"

7.1.11 Colisepsis report by veterinarian Dr. Schrader

Infections resistant to treatment such as parvovirus or colisepsis were healed with the commensurate infusions.

The complete report can be found under "Parvovirus" by veterinarian Dr. Schrader.

7.1.12 Intestinal infections
according to veterinarian Dr. Schrader

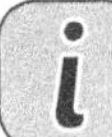

Intestinal infections

With infections of the airway or the intestinal tract bring 1 - 2 drops of 22.5% sodium chlorite solution into contact with 1 - 2 drops of 3.5% hydrochloric acid solution for precisely 1 minute (preferably use a common shot glass), and by means of a syringe add approximately 2 - 5 mL (0.068 - 0.169 fl oz) tap water, stir, draw the mix up into the syringe and administer the mixture directly into the jaw of the animal (best sideways into the cheek pouch). This treatment should be undertaken after feeding, and never on an empty stomach! In extreme cases administer twice daily. Here too, no harm to the patient has been observed on any occasion.

7.1.13 Diarrhea and epilepsy

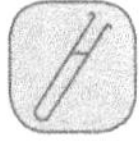

Treatment

On the first day a 65 kg (143,300 lb) Saint Bernard was given 8 drops of CDS 6 times directly into the mouth. By evening the stool was already visibly firmer and the indications of gastritis had disappeared. In addition he received a teaspoon each of bentonite and zeolite, and for his general condition OPC (oligomeric proanthocyanidin) to follow up on the treatment with CDS. CDS was again administered 3 times daily; the dose was subsequently increased by 2 drops per day. In that the patient was a Saint Bernard, the dosage was increased up to 20 drops 3 times daily. Based on her own instincts the owner halted the medication on the second day. After a few days I received a call, she said that it was wonderful to have a new dog and that she could cheerfully look to a positive future for the dog. As he became at times agitated he unfortunately suffered another attack. As the risk was high, selected calming and bolstering plant-based tinctures were prescribed.

7.1.14 Eczema, weeping

Description practical example:

My dog was stung behind the ear, assailant unknown. Initially I waited a week, but the swelling grew and grew. I then found my way to a veterinarian and received antibiotics for the dog. After a week it burst, pus came out and the swelling subsided. We thought all was now fine, but two days later it began to swell up again. So I went back to the veterinarian to shed light on the diagnosis; the dog received another antibiotic shot and the wound was rinsed. I treated the area as instructed with ca-lendula tincture and salve - it looked good now as there was discharge and there was hardly any swelling. Another two days and the area was inflamed (red and hot) yet again.

We decided to dab on the surface the swelling with MMS and DMSO, morning and evenings.

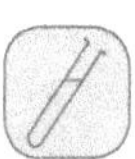

Treatment

Following two days of regular dabbing on of MMS with MSO morning and evening, I then administered 1 drop of activated MMS (the bitch weighs 11 kg/24.250 lb) twice daily. The bump soon burst and a hole of round 0.5 cm (0.1.968 in) appeared in the skin, which was to be expected as already one week earlier this wound could be seen. The dispensation of MMS and DMSO two times a day, internally and orally, continued. Within four days the wound had healed and only clean fluid came from the wound, unlike the previous times. Soon the wound was completely healed. All's well that ends well! Mission accomplished!

Treatment: 1 drop MMS activated with activator and water 2 times daily.

7.1.15 Eczema

Description practical example:

A Leonberger, one and half years old at the time, was an enthusiastic swimmer.
After bathing I discovered a 10 cm (3.937 in) wide, itchy, weeping sore behind the right ear.

The following treatment was prescribed:

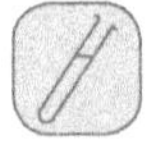

Treatment

I sprayed on a liberal amount of undiluted CDS thrice daily and then dabbed gently with a paper towel. I allowed this to dry a while and spread aloe vera gel on (the dog felt no itch, so there was no problem with his scratching at the wound, which often hinders healing).

The area dried appreciably, the redness had faded away after two days, and from day 3 to day 5 I treated the spot one or two times each day with undiluted CDS.

I did this as a precaution to disinfect. The drying with paper towel was no longer required. I continued to apply the aloe vera gel.

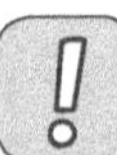

Important! Although CDS is very much weaker and gentler than MMS, it can also be somewhat corrosive in large amounts. To spray was in this case fine, though for mouthwash a half bottle of CDS is certainly excessive. Please take care when administering CDS.

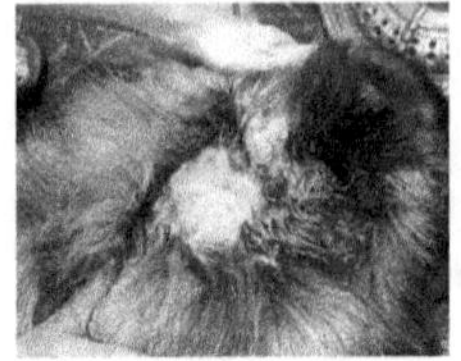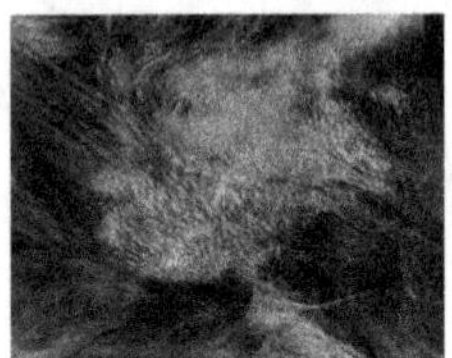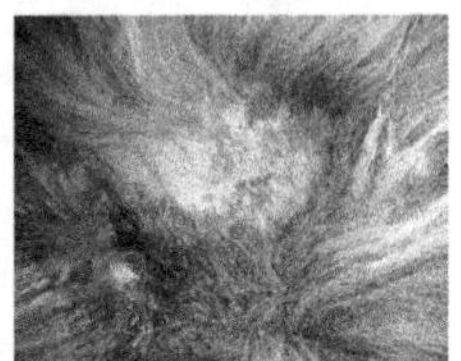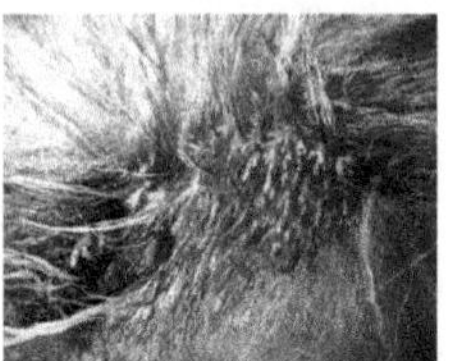

Day 1 to day 5

7.1.16 Eczema on the skin

Description practical example:

A Doberman of approximately 34 kg (74.957 lb) was a patient at my practice. She suffered from skin eczema and boils, and was passed from doctor to doctor for two years. She was even operated on, which was entirely unhelpful.

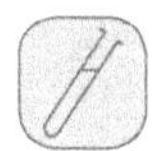

Treatment

The dog underwent Bioresonance therapy three times a day. The owner administered 4 drops of CDS in water directly in the mouth 3 times daily. The wounds were sprayed with a MMS solution as well. One week later, the wounds had closed and the skin healed (See: Photographs).

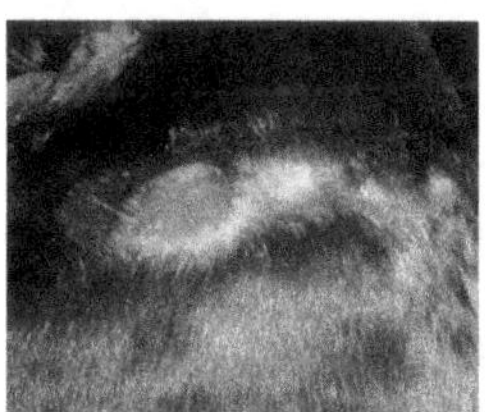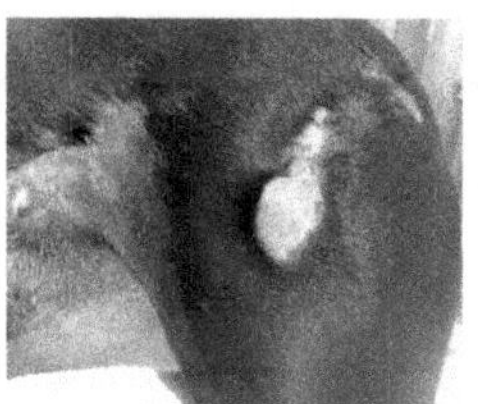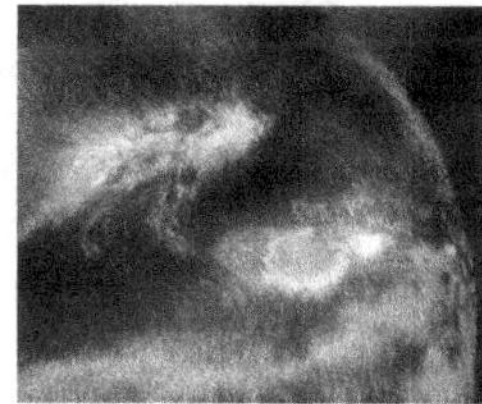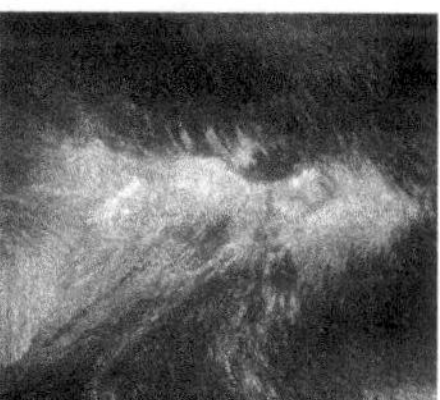

7.1.17 Eczema on the nose

Description practical example, report by Susanne R.:

Suna, a Galgo, from Borken, approximately 28 kg (61.729 lb), had eczema on the nose.

The owner had tried many things (veterinarian), but nothing brought tangible results.

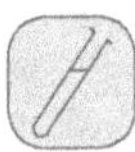

Treatment

The area was dabbed a number of times daily with MMS (2 drops activated in a shot glass, then topped up with water) for about three weeks. The area healed well and the problem has not reoccurred (See: Photographs).

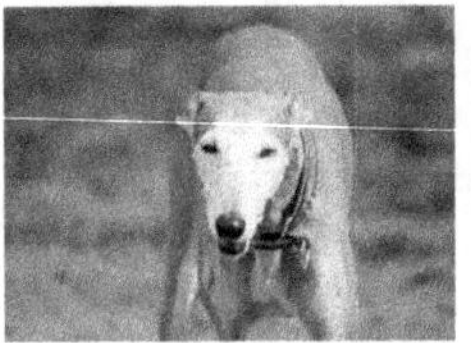 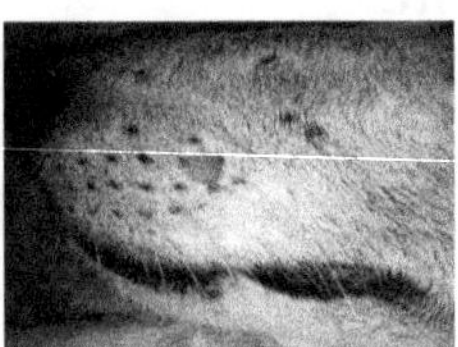 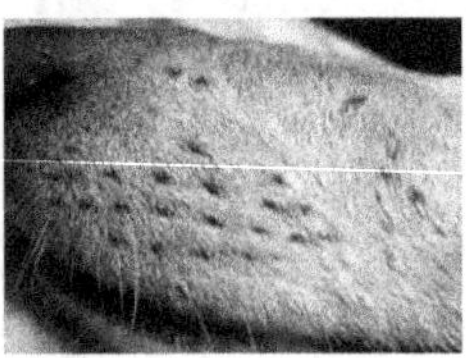 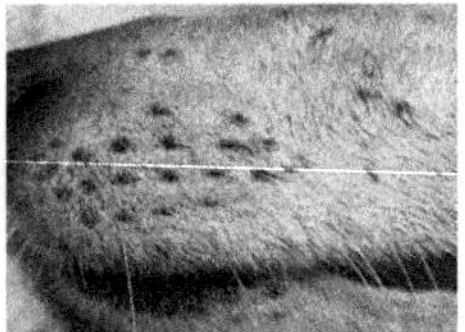

7.1.18 Inflammation on the leg

Description practical example, report by Susanne R.:
Scotty, a small crossbreed, had an inflammation on the leg. I bathed the paws with MMS to begin and then rubbed in MMS/ DMSO daily. Evenings I applied milking grease with marigold tea. The rub-on mixture was similar to the following spray, but without the aloe vera essence.

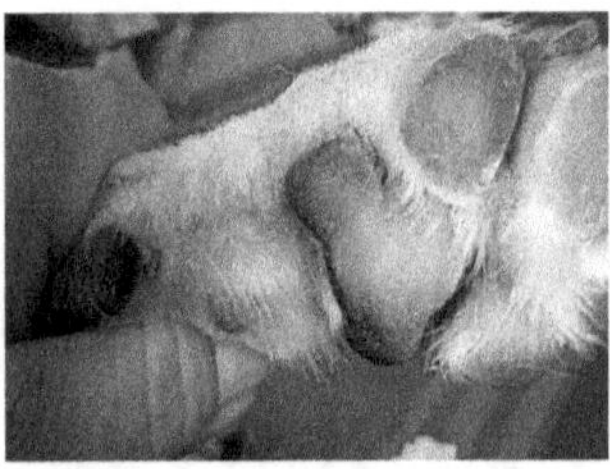 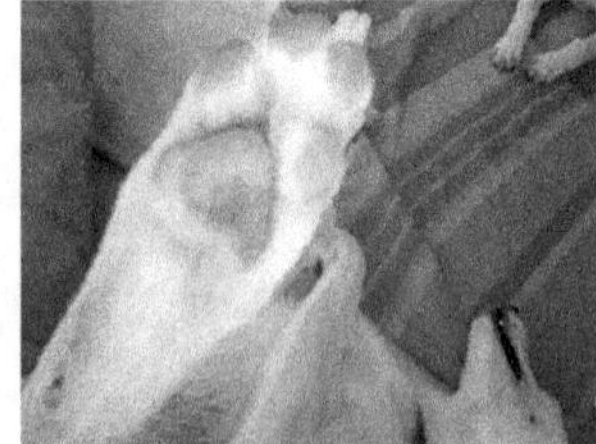

Before

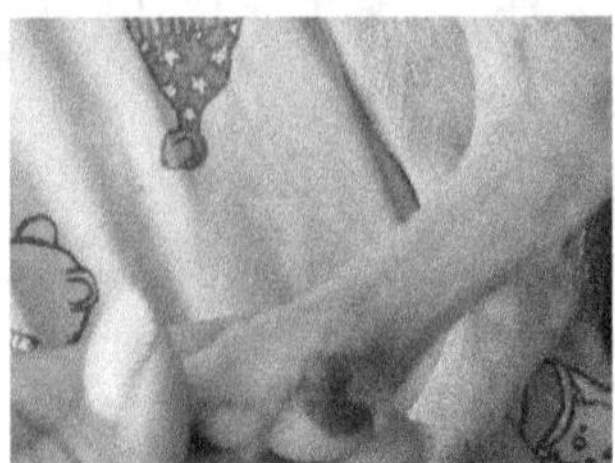 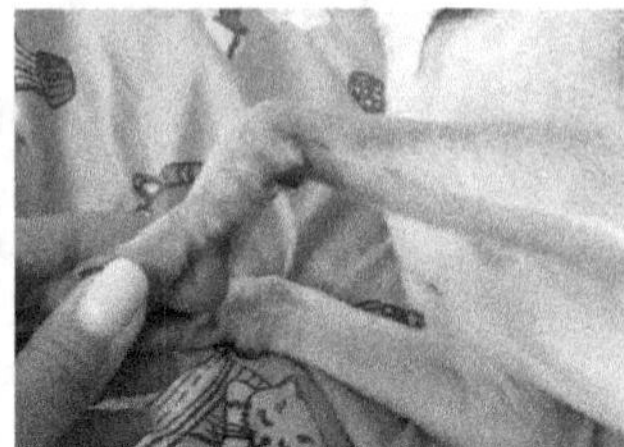

After: The fur grew back.

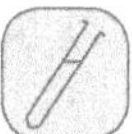

Treatment

4 drops MMS + activator, 4 drops DMSO, 15 mL (0.507 fl oz) aloe vera essence,
10 mL (0.338 fl oz) water; spray on 3 to 4 times daily and rub in aloe vera essence
for 4 days.

After four days the inflammation was healed (See: photographs
above p. 164).

7.1.19 Epilepsy and diarrhea

See: 7.1.13

7.1.20 Vomiting

Description practical example:
I received an emergency call from a woman one Saturday evening. Her three-year-old bitch had vomited copiously for two
hours following the evening meal. She had been retching continually for an hour, while her stomach convulsed violently.

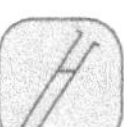

Treatment

We activated 2 drops of MMS and diluted it with 10 mL (0.338 fl oz) of water.
The solution was then sprayed directly into the mouth. After only 15 minutes
the stomach was calmed and the retching had stopped.

The dog ran about for a while. That passed gradually, and after
another 30 minutes she lay down to sleep. In the morning she
was her old self, and food tasted good again.

7.1.21 Fever

Description practical example:

An older crossbreed bitch (approx. 23 kg/50.706 lb) with fever received an antibiotic and cortisone. Subsequent to a conversation with the veterinarian the medications were discontinued, as there were no signs of improvement.

Unfortunately the owner did not carry on with the treatment, and shortly the drama started from the beginning. Afterwards there was cause for suspicion that the owner was subject to the Munchhausen proxy syndrome.

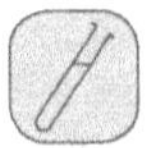

Treatment

On day one she was given 1 drop of MMS in water hourly approx. 5 times. The dose was administered directly into the mouth by means of a syringe.
The second day the dosage was increased to 2 drops each hour. From the third day on 2 drops were dispensed 3 times daily. After a week the dog was finally, and for the first time, free of fever.

The Munchhausen Syndrome

The Munchhausen proxy syndrome is a psychic disorder by which the person affected feigns the symptoms of being ill. For example: There is a case of a city-woman who stabbed herself in the leg and rushed to a nearby medical practice claiming she had been attacked. With Munchhausen syndrome the feigned illness or injury is projected onto a child entrusted to the caregiver, or onto a pet in some cases! The person affected by Munchhausen syndrome administers tablets or the like to the child or animal in order to evoke symptoms of illness, calls upon a doctor or veterinarian thereby gaining attention, and then feels rewarded for his/her ministrations.

7.1.22 Fever and autoimmune disorder

Description practical example:

A ten-year-old male Kangal (approx. 52 kg/114.640 lb) was given up for dead. The dog was born with an autoimmune disorder, meaning that he had all his life received strong medication with powerful side effects. In spite of this all had gone well for him until quite recently he all of a sudden one day had a 40 °C (104 ° F) fever. He was immediately taken to the animal clinic where he was treated for five days and then discharged free of fever. His condition was to be sure afebrile, though he was listless and his bladder simply drained without pressure. There was another side effect: The treatment cost Euro 1,600 (approx. USD 1800). When the owner requested a report from the clinic she received the sobering news that none existed. Nevertheless, eleven tablets to be dispensed morning and evening over the next two days were provided as follow up treatment.

The fever reappeared however when the tablets were finished. On top of that, changes to the liver were discerned.

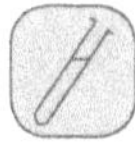

Treatment

The following was administered:
Day 1: 5 drops MMS + activator + approx. 10 mL (0.338 fl oz) apple juice, 7 times
Day 2 + 3: 5 drops MMS + activator + approx. 10 mL (0.338 f oz) apple juice, 2 times

The fever disappeared, the dog's mood was cheerful, and he ran about happy and frisky. Talk of the imminent end or his being put to sleep is no more.

The dosage for this dog was comparatively high - it was specifically adjusted to his purposes. Note: Use this dosage only after case-specific testing!

7.1.23 Mouth odor

Description practical example, report by Eva W.:
"Our dog had bad breath.

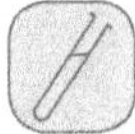

Treatment

Add 5 - 10 drops CDS to the water receptacle, repeating until the odor is gone."

"Our cat too - probably because it was the dog bowl – indulged: it would have been 1 - 3 or so drops of CDS. Animals sense when they are in need of something and when it does them good."

7.1.24 Giardi parasites

Description practical example:
The owner was growing disconsolate as result of an endless and expensive odyssey from veterinarian to veterinarian that brought no improvement for a twenty-kilogram (44.092 lb) dog. The dog's diarrhea was getting worse not better, and its general condition was no longer good.

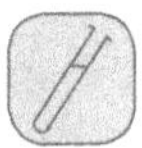

Treatment

We commenced the treatment with 3 drops of MMS + activator + some water mixed with the food, two times daily.

Already after one day the stool became paste like, and firm the next day.

The dog is visibly in good spirits again. He has been free of symptoms and complaints for a year. Thank you!

7.1.25 Grass mites

Description practical example:

The patient was a two-year-old female with grass mites, principally at the base of the tail and the anus.

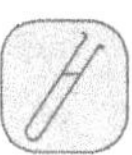

Treatment

We washed her with a mixture of 20 drops of MMS (activated) and approximately 5 Liter (1.320 gal) of water. As the dog was longhaired, I advised the owner to wipe her down with a cotton cloth (an old diaper) in the open air. Following the third wash we could already see how the mites detached themselves and the reddened skin brought on by the constant scratching was again pink. The dog also ingested MMS due to her licking herself after being washed.

7.1.26 Skin infection
according to veterinarian Dr. Schrader

"Chlorine dioxide synthesized by us has long been deployed with 100% success, especially when treating skin infections, and without any harm to patients:

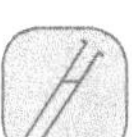

Treatment

For this purpose 20 drops of 22.5% sodium chlorite solution are mixed with 20 drops of 3.5% hydrochloric acid and dissolved in 60 mL (2.028 fl oz) cold tap water for exactly 1 minute. On account of the poisonous nature of the gases discharged, production should take place under local exhaust ventilation, or alternatively, next to an open window.

Dabbing the infected regions of skin with this solution (a more intensive action takes place with prior treatment using 50% DMSO solution) results in the instantaneous elimination of all accessible microorganisms. For good measure the application should be repeated a number of times.

In cases of skin inflammation brought on by allergies, parallel treatment with cortisones and/or antihistamines may, where appropriate, transpire.

7.1.27 Hot Spots

Description practical example:
Description practical example:
A Bulldog-cross had many hot spots on his back and on the root of his tail, some were open. In spite of numerous visits to the veterinarian entailing repeated administration of cortisone and antibiotics there was no visible improvement. The veterinarian could not offer an accurate diagnosis regarding the bacteria.

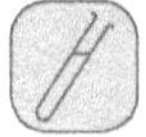

Treatment

"We began treatment with CDS. It was our last hope. We medicated internally and externally.
I unfortunately no longer know the exact dosage. What can I say? After three months the horrific episode was over. It has all healed beautifully and the dog now has marvelous fur - even one year later! No more hot spots have appeared. I can only recommend this to everyone!"

7.1.28 Castration, male

Description practical example:
A client asked what to do as a precautionary measure before and after the castration of her dog.

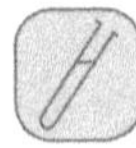

Treatment

I suggested a homeopathic medication (Nux Vomica) for the run-up. Subsequent to the operation we employed zeolite: 1 teaspoon mixed in water, added to the morning and evening meals. In addition, the wound was swabbed with CDS and DMSO (See: 6.4.8 Standard instructions wounds general). No problems arose; the wound closed after a few days without further difficulties and without antibiotics.

7.1.29 Cancer of the liver

The patient is a dog, six years old and of approximately 23 kg (50.706 lb). He came with the diagnosis of cancer of the liver that had already spread widely. The dog had visible tumors on the belly as well. He was considered by the veterinarian to be beyond treatment and ready to be put down before long.

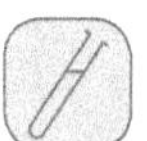

Treatment

He was fed light, raw food, without cereals. Then medicines such as Swedish bitters, apricot kernels and a mistletoe tincture, along with CDS: 8 drops 3 times daily increasing each day to attain 20 drops.

At the end of a week the owner detected visible improvement in his general state of health. Two weeks further on the nodes on the belly were smaller.

In addition he received homeopathic medications plus food supplements. The treatment with CDS continued with short pauses. Blood values slowly improved.

After almost a year his heart gave up however and he crossed the rainbow bridge.

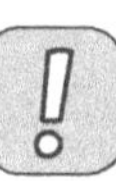

With every cancer case there is a point of no return (See: Chapter 13), for our animals as well. At this stage it is no longer important which treatment and medicines are employed: There is no triumph that evolution cannot reverse. This goes for conventional as well as alternative medicine!

7.1.30 Cirrhosis of the liver - liver inflammation - hepatitis

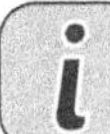

Cirrhosis of the liver - liver inflammation - hepatitis

Phenotype: Except for jaundice there was no typical set of observable characteristics, rather asymptomatic acute stage disturbance of the overall condition, listlessness, loss of appetite, disability, unwillingness to move, rheumatic discomfort, gastrointestinal problems, and fever. Urine sparse and dark in color; the stool soft, pale, clay colored. The region of the liver sensitive to pressure.

Causes: Infections from viruses, bacteria, fungus, as well as parasites and poisons.

Description practical example:

A dog (approx. 23 kg/50.706 lb) diagnosed with cirrhosis of the liver was brought to the practice. The prognosis by the veterinarian offered no hope. The dog was, so to say, beyond therapy. The problem signaled that both dog and owner were extremely sensitive and delicate.

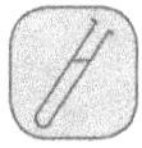

Treatment

In that the dog was clogged-up with phlegm and as a result vomited when dispensed with only 2 drops of CDS, I next treated the symptoms with homeopathy. We began with 4 drops of CDS in water and rubbed this onto the body to circumvent more vomiting (this was easy as the dog was short-haired). The medicine entered the bloodstream via the skin and was thus more tolerable.

The dog responded well, and with the incipient improvement of its general condition the internal treatment could now slowly begin with the administration of 2 drops of CDS in 10 mL (0.338 fl oz) water direct in the mouth. The treatment is ongoing.

7.1.31 Canine leishmaniosis - Mediterranean disease

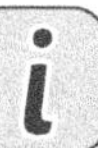

Mediterranean disease

This medical condition mostly afflicts dogs that come from southern lands such as Greece and Spain.

It is transmitted by the bite of infected sandflies. The parasites enter the bloodstream in this way.

Phenotype: Indications are inflammation of the liver, kidneys, skin, eyes, and bones.

Description, dog Pacorro with leishmaniosis:

I received an emergency call. A dog, eight months of age, approximately 14 kg (30.864 lb), with confirmed leishmaniosis (Tita over 800) ought, in the opinion of the veterinarian, be put to sleep. He was consequently turned out from the foster home and taken to another. A new placement was now urgently being sought and I was called. So we took the little fellow in. He had been administered an enormous amount of medication by the veterinarian: Heart medicine, an antirheumatic, pain relievers, leishmaniosis medicine (Allopurinol), and more.

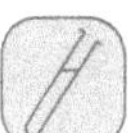

Treatment

Firstly, he was put on a raw meat diet (BARF), which suited him well. He was fed Spirulina in addition. Then came the treatment. Incidentally: All medications were called to a halt from day one.

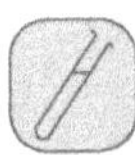

Continuation: Treatment

Day 1: 2 drops of MMS 6 times (following the final dose there was a light, short-term gagging). In addition, 2 drops of MMS were diluted in 300 mL (10.144 fl oz) of water, and the eye, which was weeping a little, was wiped.

Day 2: 2 drops of MMS 3 times.
On this day the auricles (the external part or pinna of the ear), that were somewhat reddened, were rubbed. The dog went along with everything gladly, and had fun and energy.

Day 3: 3 drops of MMS 3, times daily + arnica.

Day 4: 3 drops of MMS, 3 times daily; thin stool, light gagging in the evening.

Day 5: 2 drops of MMS 3 times daily.

Day 6: 2 drops of MMS 3 times daily.

Day 7: Pause, no MMS - plant based tincture.

Day 8: 2 drops of MMS 2 times daily; continue 2 drops of MMS, 2 times daily.

From day 9 a pause was taken, and then one teaspoon of zeolite was dispensed in the evening for one week.

Then, one teaspoon of bentonite in the morning for one week.
Additionally, from day 9: A half teaspoon of borax with magnesium (See: "Borax" Chapter 8.7) morning and evening for one week.

Then a 16 day rest.

Subsequently, 2 drops of MMS 2 times daily, and in the evening 1 teaspoon of zeolite and selenium for one week. This was specially developed for him.

After only six weeks there has been no more evidence of leishmaniosis. The dog is steadily putting on weight, is energetic and playful as should be the case for a young dog.

To stabilize, and as a precaution: 1 mL CDS (0.033 fl oz) and ½ mL (0.0169 fl oz) DMSO was administered 2 times daily for one week.

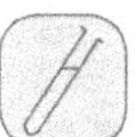

Continuation: Treatment

After approximately four months the blood values were significantly improved (Tita just over 400), and he was castrated (this should be carefully considered for subsequent to castration a recurrence of leishmaniosis is likely). After that he was given Terrakraft to strengthen the liver and kidneys; concurrently we returned to treating him with MMS as follow-up to the operation.

Here he received 3 drops of MMS + 3 drops of DMSO + approximately 50 mL (1.690 fl oz) water 3 times daily for one week. Since then there have been no signs of leishmaniosis.

7.1.32 Leishmaniosis treatment with Gefeu (general)

Treatment of leishmaniosis with
Gefeu, report from Sylke G.:

"I treated the dog's leishmaniosis with Gefeu and DMSO. Correct diet is I believe also important, and I recommend changing over to BARF (biologically appropriate raw food). In addition I dispensed MSM (methylsulfonylmethane) and, when necessary, homeopathic medicine. This must be compatible though with each animal. Most important: All of this is without Allopurinol!"

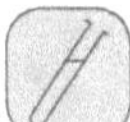

Treatment

Gefeu is dispensed 25 drops 3 times daily. Begin with 5 drops of Gefeu and increase gradually.

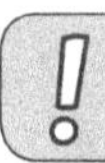

Definitely take note of the side effects of Allopurinol! Why does an animal need an anti-gout preparation, a cardiac agent, a painkiller, and the others that often come in association?

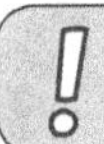

Allopurinol sinks the uric acid value and is for this reason to be used with caution, especially in cases of dogs with kidney ailments. Among the potential side effects of Allopurinol are allergic reactions, nausea, vomiting, formation of blood disorders, cultivation of kidney stones, and damage to the liver.

7.1.33 Leishmaniosis

Description practical example, report by Susanne R.:
"Micky, a female dog, roughly 8 kg (17.636 lb), arrived one Saturday evening assisted by an animal welfare association.
A veterinarian had diagnosed leishmaniosis.
According to the vet she was to be fed Allupurinol one time per day."

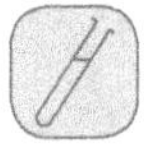

Treatment

"Instead I began immediately administering 2 drops of MMS + activator + 20 mL (0.676 fl oz) water 2 times daily, directly into the mouth. The following Thursday, i.e., after four days, she received 2 drops of MMS activated and diluted in water **hourly.**

The evening of that day she had a little cough. On Friday she received 2 drops of activated MMS in water 2 times and a soupçon of zeolite in the evening for one week.

The abdominal region and the ear were both inflamed and in parts open. I dabbed a solution consisting of 2 drops of activated MMS and 2 drops of DMSO diluted in 50 mL (1.690 fl oz) in water."

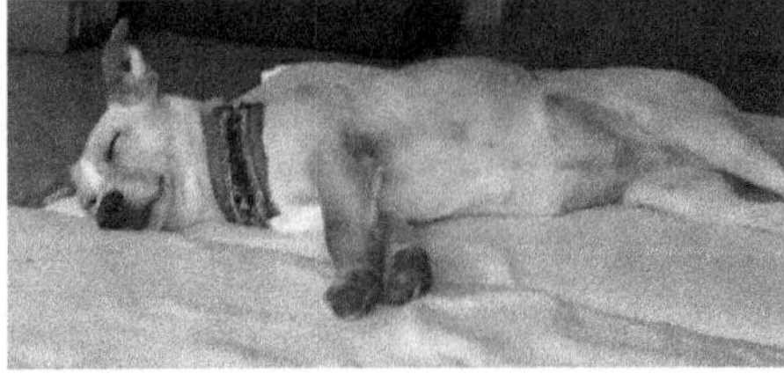

"It all healed well, and there have been no repeat episodes."

One can see here how the abdomen has healed.

7.1.34 Cutaneous leishmaniosis, open ear

Description practical example:

A dog weighing 18 kg (39.683 lb) was brought to the practice suffering from an open ear. The owner had already been through a bit. Antibiotics were out of the question, he had the feeling they had just made things worse.

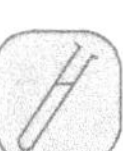

Treatment

I advised him to prepare a solution of 6 drops of MMS + activator in a glass of water, dip in a cotton cloth, and then gingerly lay this on the ear and hold it in place for one or two minutes. In the evening came a herbal salve that would soak in overnight. This was for one week, then two or three times per week. In addition he received a suitable homeopathic medicine and orally was administered 2 drops of activated MMS with water three times daily.

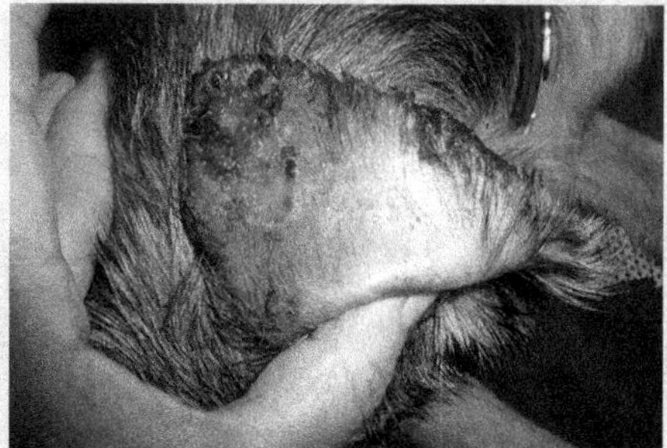

First day

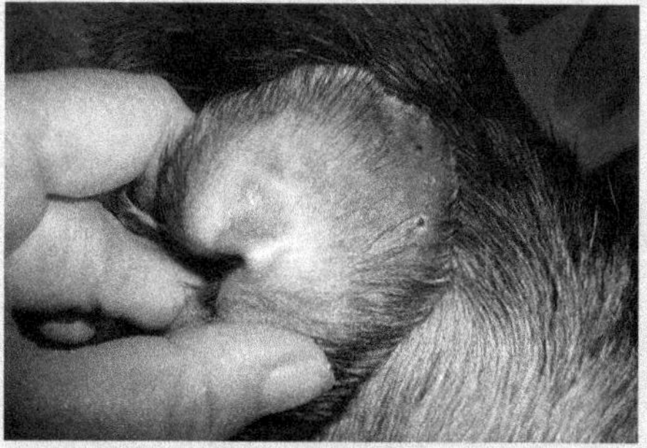

At the end of approximately four weeks

In course of the treatment I suggested a blood test as I suspected leishmaniosis, which was the case unfortunately. Though tested as positive, the Tita was, thank goodness, low. This was cutaneous leishmaniosis, also known as tropical sore. It manifests in the form of open ears and other skin problems.

As a precaution 2 drops of activated MMS with water, two times daily for 2 weeks. The ears remained free of wounds and no other skin problems appeared.

7.1.35 Lipoma on the underbelly

Description practical example:

The owner of a dog (approx. 7 kg/15.432 lb) with a number of lipoma on the underbelly rang. The dog as a puppy had had bad experiences with humans and consequently would not allow the veterinarian to handle him. It would be necessary to anesthetize it in order to perform an examination. Because the owner preferred to avoid this she came to me. Seeing that the lipoma lay under the skin and could be moved we proceeded with a simple treatment using CDS to begin.

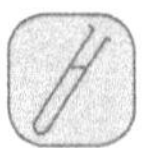

Treatment

8 drops of CDS with approx. 10 mL (0.338 fl oz) water was ingested once daily and in addition the areas were dabbed with18 drops of CDS mixed in a glass of water.

The treatment was very successful. The lipoma gradually retreated and finally dissipated.

7.1.36 Malignant lymphoma

Report by veterinarian Dr. Schrader

"In dealing with infections of the airways or the intestines we bring 1 - 2 drops of a 22.5% sodium chlorite solution together with 1 - 2 drops of 3.5% hydrochloric acid solution for exactly 1 minute (preferably use a common shot glass). By means of a syringe add 2 - 5 mL (0.068 - 0.169 fl oz) tap water, disperse the mixture, draw it back into the syringe, and administer directly into the animal's mouth (into the cheek pouch where possible); 2 times daily in critical situations. This treatment follows feeding (never on an empty stomach!) Here too, no harm to the patient has been perceived at any time. Therapy resistant infections such as parvovirus and coli-sepsis can be healed with the corresponding infusions as well. Interestingly, between 2013 and the present day we have been able to terminate seven cases of malignant lymphoma in dogs with this oral method."

The complete report can be read under "Parvovirus" by veterinarian Dr. Schrader.

7.1.37 Mites

Description practical example:
The patient was a female Dachshund mix that had for two years suffered from recurring mite attacks. The veterinarians could make no progress, the infestation of the ears occurred over and over. The whole animal medicine cabinet was sampled - without success. The veterinarian's explanation was that the dog's auditory canals were too narrow.

The poor mouse was plagued nonstop; constant scratching and whimpering were the outcome.
The full report can be found under "Parvovirus."

Treatment 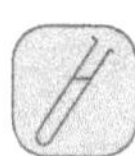

The following mixture was applied:

100 mL (3.381 fl oz) water + 20 drops of CDS.

This solution was sprayed into the ears daily and massaged in. After eight days the problem was a thing of the past.

7.1.38 Multiresistant germs

See: "Ear - Multiresistant germs"

7.1.39 Open areas

Description practical example:
The Leonberger Max (over 50 kg/110.231 lb) was four years old when he came to me. The veterinarians could not help, always had antibiotics on offer, but unfortunately no cure. Max had 6 to 8 open wounds, some as big as a fist, distributed over his body. Following countless doses of antibiotics his general condition continued to deteriorate and there was talk of putting him down!

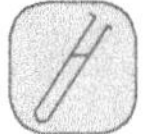

Treatment

His diet was modified to being chemical free, species appropriate and wholefood. Detoxifying medicines commensurate with his special needs and MMS were administered orally and externally. After three weeks Max was almost back to his old self but for one area that healed after few days more. He is now well on the way and finds joy in life!

MMS internal:
The dose was specifically matched to the needs of this animal. As you can see the amounts are unlike those dispensed to other dogs of similar weight:
A mixture of 4 drops MMS and activator in a glass of water was prepared, then a ½ glass added to his meal 2 times daily.

MMS external:
Prepare a mix of 10 drops activated MMS and 500 mL (16.907 fl oz) water, and 2 - 3 times each day dab this on the open wounds, which act as valves to dispose of poisons.

7.1.40 Open wound, presumably a bite

Description practical example:

Asco, a Golden Retriever from Borken, had a wound on the side that would not heal.

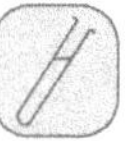

Treatment

The owner cleaned the said region several times a day with MMS - this area is no longer to be located. Two drops of activated MMS were put in a shot glass (2 cl/0.338 fl oz), which was then topped up with water. The lesion healed with every day and was gone in a week.

Side effects: The fur became more beautiful!

7.1.41 Ear, multiresistant germs

Description practical example:

The patient was a dog with multiresistant germs in one ear; no antibiotic could help as these germs had developed resistance.

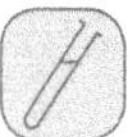

Treatment

I rinsed the ear out 2 times daily with 1 drop of MMS in 15 mL (0.507 fl oz) water. Even these germs had no choice but to disappear.

7.1.42 Ear inflammation, chronic

Description practical example:

"My French Bulldog suffered chronic ear inflammation. One ear was again in good order, while the other was appreciably better after daily administration of CDS.

Since I have administered CDS my dogs again sleep the night through, their smell has changed, and their fur shines gorgeously and is very soft.

I have now begun the same with my cats. They reacted to CDS by vomiting copiously - mostly they rejected larger amounts of fluid that appeared to be water-like. I will now simply dispense smaller doses. The dogs receive 5 drops mixed in water. I drip some CDS and water in their ears as well: 5 drops in water twice daily. The cats get 1 - 2 drops (reduced dosage) in their drinking water daily. I am curious to see how it all progresses. The dogs and the cats are all top fit."

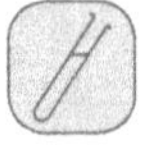

Treatment

Dogs: 5 drops of CDS in water

Cats: 1 - 2 drops of CDS in the drinking water

7.1.43 Earache

Description practical example:
The veterinarian's diagnosis was an ear inflammation. By means of animal communication the male dog (17 kg/37.478 lb) pointed out the root cause as being toothache and inflammation of the upper jaw (maxilla).

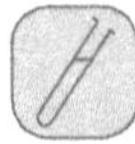

Treatment

We medicated with a thyme tincture and CDS, orally and above the auditory canal. Procedure: 12 drops CDS 3 times daily for 2 weeks, plus a solution of 12 drops CDS in 10 mL (0.338 fl oz) of water in a bottle dispensed one drop at a time with the aid of a pipette into the ear many times a day.

At the end of one week he was free of pain; following the treatment there was no recurrence of the inflammation.

7.1.44 Otitis externa -
inflammation of the outer auditory canal

Long-eared dog breeds are predestined to be affected by ear inflammation. Grime, dust, foreign bodies (insects), mites, bacteria and fungi can collect and bring about inflammation in this warm and humid system of canals.

Description practical example:

A very sensitive Rottweiler was a patient at my practice. He was often afflicted with inflammation of the ears and the veterinarian had no fix. I learned via animal communication that the trigger was a tick bite. After consulting with the owner, who confirmed that it had been bitten by a tick, the treatment commenced.

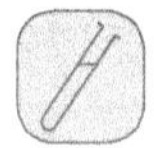

Treatment

The owner prepared a glass of water with 12 drops of CDS and cleaned the ear using a cotton swab. Since then our "sensitive one" has had hardly a problem, and when a symptom appears there is always MMS at hand.

7.1.45 Parvovirus

Parvovirus report from Hungary
by an animal shelter owner:

As a result of the conversation with Frank about Moringa oleifera and CDS I became curious. Seeing that I already had 13 dogs I wanted to test it so I ordered CDS to try that first, not without success.

I then tried it on my little Dachshund-cross. Her history of suffering was already almost two years long.

The veterinarians got nowhere; again and again she got mites in her ears. Bottom line: The animal medical dispensary was exhausted and soon after the dog had the same problem. The doctor's response was that the dog's auditory canals were too narrow. The poor mouse, constantly plagued, incessantly scratched and whimpered.

So by my own hand I mixed a CDS solution: 20 drops CDS in 100 mL (3.381 fl oz) water. I sprayed this daily into the ears then massaged it in, after eight days the malady was a thing of the past.

I had further success with the up to 99% deadly parvovirus. I have already saved the lives of four dogs in all thanks to treatment with CDS. My veterinarians presented me with a hair-raising scenario: That, at the time of the initial outbreak, courtesy of a whelp from the Nagikanisza Animal Home, I brought the pestilence with me.

It would infect all the animals, twelve at the time, and it would be dreadful, I was harshly told. In my initial despair I wrote Frank asking how many drops and how much water I should use. His answer 100 mL (3.381 fl oz) water and 10 drops of CDS dispensed hourly. There you go, the little mouse Susi survived the virus. All the rooms were disinfected each day, cleaned and sprayed with a solution of 200 mL (6.762 fl oz) water plus 40 drops of CDS. The cushions and blankets were burned. In that dogs live in packs there was a great danger that the vet may have been correct.

Still uncertain whether the medicine would really hold to its promise, and as a precaution against contagion I put, and continue to do so, 3 drops of CDS in the water containers of the other furry-noses.

After eight days the whole thing was of the past. None of the pack of furry-noses was infected - I am most thankful to Frank for this medicine.

In the meantime I have treated 4 whelps that had parvovirus with CDS; all survived and none of my 16 dogs was infected. So: I swear by CDS.

Another illness happened to one of my furry-noses. What it was exactly, I don't know. She had fever and a cough, maybe kennel cough, I can't really say. Because I had CDS I began to treat the furry-nose with that for three days: She has no more fever and the cough is gone, thanks to CDS."

7.1.46 Rubber eraser nose

Treatment

"We made a solution of 6 drops of MMS, activator and a glass of water, and using a cloth lightly rubbed it on the nose once daily. Then came a herbal salve (Hamamelis) on the nose. Now it is smooth and shining."

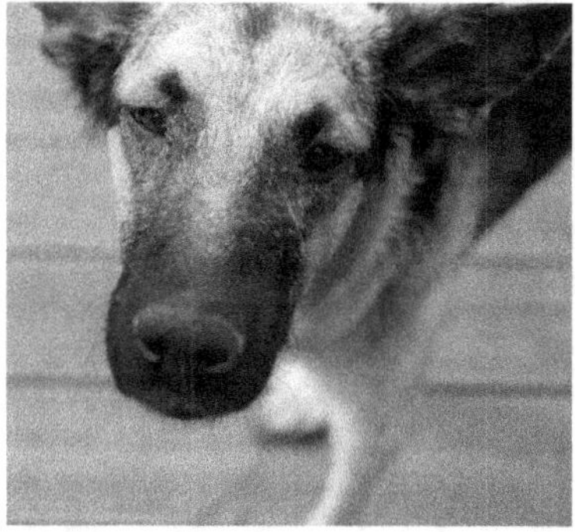

Before

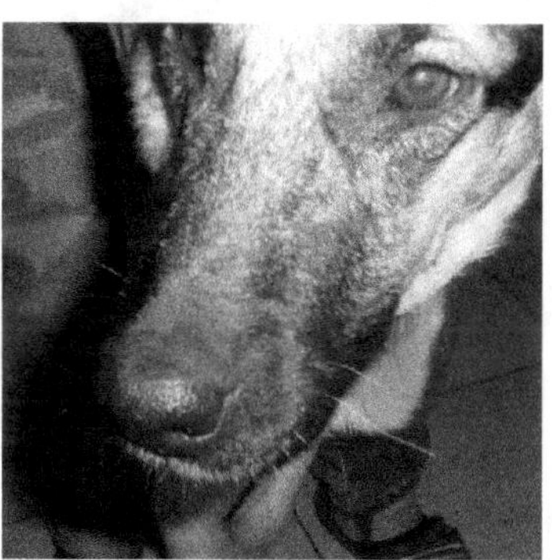

After

7.1.47 Canine distemper

Description practical example,
report by Sylke Georgoulis:

" I received a dog, Lotte, about six months old, completely inoculated (the full program!), and already castrated from animal welfare. The veterinarian confirmed that now she had distemper (despite vaccination!) - in his view there was no chance of recovery.

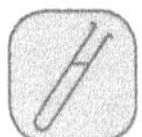

Treatment

I tried homeopathic medicines on the little mouse, and dispensed Gefeu along with MMS. Unfortunately, I no longer know the dosage.

One year on, Lotte is very well and enjoys the best of health."

7.1.48 Stray dog

Description practical example, report by Leo Koehof:
"I have two lovely photos for your book. I gathered up this dog from the side of the road in Africa eight weeks ago. Most like-

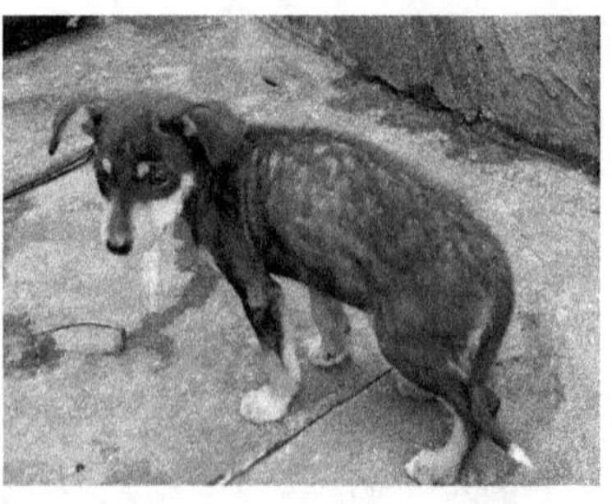
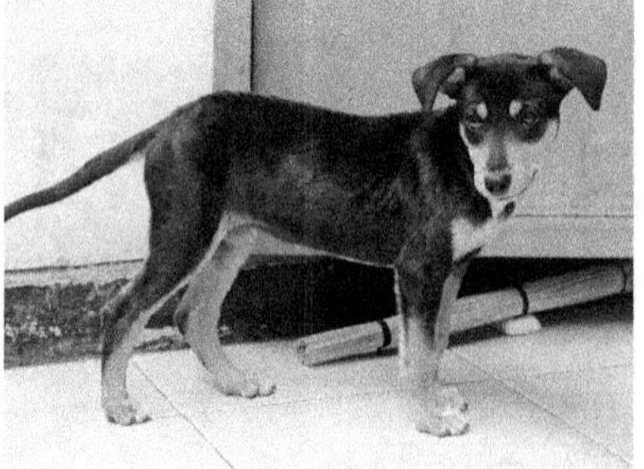

ly he would otherwise no longer be alive. I gave him MMS daily, and an overdose one time in the week to deworm him. In addition I sprayed his skin with MMS Gold daily. I fed him milk with raw egg, moringa powder and zeolite.

We then began with meat and meat broth. The second photo is four weeks after commencing treatment. People from the neighborhood came to see him. They had never seen such a pretty dog. Even a dog breeder came by, but that was on the day I had to fly back. The next time I will explain how one brings dogs up to be so healthy and strong.

I'll keep you informed.
Leo"

7.1.49 Tumor on the eyelid

Description practical example, report by Eva W.:
"From one day to the next a fast-growing malignant tumor appeared on the lower eyelid of my old bitch. This protruded half way into the eye. Using a pipette I applied 1 - 2 drops of a solution consisting of 1 - 2 drops of 50% DMSO and the same amount of CDS mixed with water to the eye. I did this exactly three times and the tumor was gone! Sounds like a miracle, but that's how it was!"

7.1.50 Tumor on the foreleg

Description practical example:
A female dog of 15 kg (33.069 lb) had already had an aggressive, fast growing tumor removed from her left foreleg three times. Nine or ten days later the tumor grew back.

It reappeared two days following the most recent operation. We then began treatment with MMS.

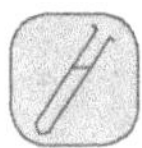

Treatment

We prepared a solution of 1 drop of MMS plus activator (1:1) and 100 mL (3.381 fl oz) water. We poured the liquid into a bottle and divided this into 10 portions that were then dispensed through the day. We increased the number of drops each day by 1 drop of MMS plus acid and water. On the 20th day, at 20 drops of MMS (daily dose) and acid, a first reaction showed up: A light gagging. Thereupon, we waited 3 days.

You will of course say that this was too much for her bodyweight. We tested with this dog and she absolutely required it. As you can read at the end of this report this was the correct procedure for her.

She received vitamins and a homeopathic medicine for the constitution as backup over the whole period. Her diet was changed to being grain free. Added to her food was a high-grade bio linseed oil for the omega 3 fatty acids.

Following the 3 day pause we continued with the 20 drops of MMS, acid and water (naturally this was also increased daily). For 30 days the treatment was kept up until we took a 5 day break before resuming with the 20 drops of MMS, acid and water split into 8 - 10 portions for another 30 days.

The doses were dispensed with a one-hour interval between the first and last meals.

The dog has been healthy for a year now!

7.1.51 Vaginal discharge, purulent

Description practical example:

A four-year-old Rottweiler-Labrador (approx. 40 kg/88,184 lb) had subsequent to being on heat, persistent, at times purulent, vaginal discharge.

Immediate castration was advised, though the uterus was normal according to the ultrasound scan.

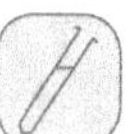

Treatment

I added 5 drops of activated MMS to approximately 100 mL (3.381 fl oz) of water or apple juice mixture and administered approximately 5 mL (0.169 fl oz) of the mix by means of a syringe 3 times daily.

Though the discharge stopped with the initial application, I dispensed the mixture for a week, reducing the rate to two times each day.

It was necessary to repeat the treatment after about a month as the symptoms reappeared.

The dog has now been free of any symptoms for nearly a year.

7.1.52 Ulcerous gums and phantom pregnancy

Description practical example:
A dog (14 kg/30.864 lb) with ulcerous gingival inflammation,
and every sign of a pseudo pregnancy.

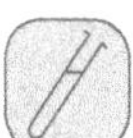

Treatment

The phantom pregnancy I treated with Bach flowers that were especially attuned to the dog. For the gums we administered CDS with approx. 20 mL (0.676 fl oz) water directly into the mouth.

Day 1: 4 drops of CDS hourly, 5 - 6 times per day.
Day 2: 8 drops of CDS hourly.
Day 3: 12 drops of CDS hourly, then 12 drops 3 times daily for a week.

After two weeks the owner telephoned. The pseudo pregnancy had normalized. The inflammation was no longer discernable. The dog was doing just fine.

7.1.53 Swollen teat

Description practical example:
A swollen teat and beneath that a swelling were noticed on a dog (approx. 32 kg/70.547 lb).
The client came directly to me as she wanted to avoid the machinery of veterinarians. We commenced the treatment with MMS that very day.

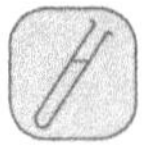

Treatment

On the first day the dog was administered 1 mL (20 drops/0.033 fl oz) of CDS 5 - 6 times mixed with water and cottage cheese. Alongside, the area was dabbed with a solution consisting of 2 mL (40 drops/0.067 fl oz) of CDS and approx. 200 mL (6.762 fl oz) water many times a day. From the second day on she was administered 2 drops of MMS, acid and water, again with a teaspoon of cottage cheese, 3 times daily. Already on the second day the swelling and the lump were not to be seen. Just to be sure, she was treated for another three days. The dog is to this day without symptoms.

7.1.54 Kennel cough

Report from an animal shelter in Hungary:
"... another occurrence of sickness afflicted my furry-noses. Exactly what it was I cannot say. The bitch had fever and a cough, maybe kennel cough, I can't be sure. Seeing that I already had CDS I used that to treat the furry-nose. Three days later she was no longer feverish and the cough was gone - thanks to CDS."

The complete report can be found under "Parvovirus."

7.2 Cat disorders that have been successfully treated with MMS

It is common knowledge that cats are difficult to treat - perhaps this is why I love these little parlor tigers and their personalities so. Some of them repeatedly call for one to come up with something new to be able to treat them; at times a trick may be necessary. Cats are very aware of what does them good and what does harm. The owner is of the utmost importance with these darlings: If she betrays fear in the preparation, worry, or only discomfort, then often cats refuse to cooperate.

> **Potential effects of dry pet food on cats**
>
> A major issue as concerns cats is the kidneys. Indications of sickness or debility relating to the kidneys are as a rule due to food. The great evil is dry pet food. Why? The cat is an inhabitant of the desert and as a rule drinks little. To process kibble they must imbibe three times the amount of water. Normally a cat takes in liquids by way of the food, the blood of a mouse for instance. When fluid intake is insufficient, uric acid is reduced due to the long span of time required for digestion; the kidneys are thus encumbered and damaged over time.

7.2.1 Afflictions of old age

Description, practical example from a client's letter:
"I currently administer Gefeu solution to my 18 year-old cat, which is extremely fastidious as regards the taste of her food, though she quaffs Gefeu drops without a fuss. She must take them for the small afflictions of old age, such as osteoarthritis, et cetera.
Already on the second day of intake, after a long interlude, she presented a mouse, and this has been repeated many times since then. I regard it as a sign of rejuvenation.

At one point I called a halt to the process, as I could find no information relating to hyperactive thyroid glands, the real problem, and administration of MMS. Now, I again give her a trace of diluted Gefeu in her food. She is rather iffy about smells, but this she quaffs, to put it nicely."

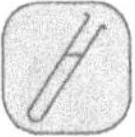

Treatment

Administer a trace of Gefeu with meals. Unfortunately no indication regarding amounts was supplied. You can apply the standard instructions in Chapter 6.

Since this time the cat comes across as livelier and more agile.

7.2.2 Inflammation of the eyes

Description practical example:
The patient was a cat with an eye inflammation. The eye wept intensively all day long.

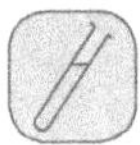

Treatment

Rinse out with 50 mL (0.169 fl oz) water containing 1 drop of activated MMS. After only two days the eye was dry, and the inflammation no longer apparent.

7.2.3 Festering eye

Description practical example:
When she was still a kitten this cat lost both eyes. Six years later she sustained a problem with an eye socket. This was sewn closed. A few months later the socket began to fester anew. That was the occasion for the owner to contact me for she did not want to overtax the cat with narcotics yet again.

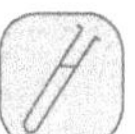

> **Treatment**
>
> For two days the cat received 2 drops of CDS 3 times daily, plus 4 drops of CDS diluted in 10 mL (0.338 fl oz) water dispensed directly into the mouth 3 times daily. She received a plant tincture in addition.

After three days the weeping was already improved, and the pain had abated. The sticky puss was then removed by the veterinarian and rinsed out. Without more narcotics, let alone another operation, it all healed well.

7.2.4 Blood in the urine

Description practical example:

I noticed blood in my cat's urine, which indicated inflammation of the bladder. The cat urinated often and without control.

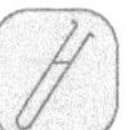

> **Treatment**
>
> Dispense 1 drop of MMS in 5 mL (0.169 fl oz) water directly into the mouth many times a day.

After only five days she was visibly healed, and exhibited no new symptoms.

7.2.5 Colon cancer

Description practical example:

The patient was a three-year-old cat with colon cancer at an early stage. According to the veterinarian there was little hope of recovery.

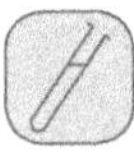

Treatment

First of all we began the therapy with a change of diet to light foods with lean, raw meat. To support the immune system and her general condition she was given Terrakraft as well as homeopathic medicines and Bach flowers.

We began the MMS therapy with a ½ drop of MMS 3 times daily over 2 days; 1 drop of MMS 3 times daily for 2 more days; then a change to CDS starting with 8 drops of CDS 3 times daily. Further increases were not necessary. She received this dose for another 4 weeks. Following two weeks there was evident improvement. The cat became more active; the change to BARF (Biologically Appropriate Raw Food Diet) was easy and very effective. At the end of 4 weeks we took a break of about 6 weeks and then resumed treatment with 8 drops of CDS 3 times daily.

After 6 months the cat seemed to be very well, so we organized a blood test: Everything was just great! Every now and then she is administered CDS as a precaution.

7.2.6 Diabetes mellitus

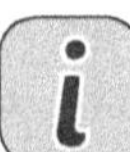

Diabetes mellitus

A chronic, festering metabolic disease

Phenotype: Incipient excess weight, unexplained weight loss, muscle weakness, loss of strength, increasing fatigue, blurred vision, changes to the fur

Causes: Overeating and malnourishment, incorrect feeding, hormonal and constitutional factors

A clarification of the cause of this condition by means of a Hemogram and urinalysis is important. What often occurs is that cats are prescribed a special dry-food. This has negative repercussions in that the metabolism and the organs are encumbered even further.

At first it was important with this seven-year-old tomcat suffering diabetes to change its diet to lean raw meat.

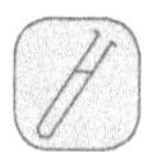

Treatment

The tom received 1 drop of activated MMS diluted with water three times daily for three days; this was increased to 2 drops daily thereafter. The treatment was complemented with herbs and Bach flowers.

At the end of two months the tom's blood levels approached normal and he was friskier than he had long been. More than a year later the values were still in the green region. Following further enquiries I learned that the tom is still full of beans.

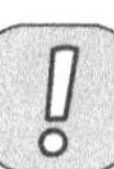

Recently I had a conversation about diabetes with a cat owner. He was confounded as to how a cat could contract diabetes when it ate no sugar. I suggested he consider the ingredients of industrially prepared cat and dog food. It is in particular important to know that sugar is at times disguised behind obscure nomenclature, and not seldom. Naturally there are other reasons for diabetes. As can be seen in the information box about diabetes mellitus, sugar plays an accessory role as a trigger. It is crucial to take nutrition overall into account.

A tomcat of around ten-years-old came to the practice diagnosed as being diabetic.

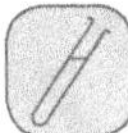

Treatment

He received goat colostrum juice, a herbal tincture, fresh stinging nettle, sage tea and Bach flowers.

In addition he received 1 drop of activated MMS diluted with approx. 10 mL (0.338 fl oz) water, three times daily for three days, increased to 2 drops daily thereafter.

The treatment suited the tom. It proved no problem to give him MMS. He tolerated it well, suffering neither diarrhea nor queasiness. This is not always so at the practice.

7.2.7 Diarrhea

Tomcat with diarrhea and regurgitation of food.

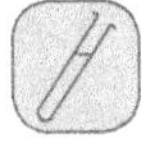

Treatment

The tom was given 1 drop of CDS with a little water 3 times daily over two weeks. The diarrhea disappeared and the regurgitation showed up only sometimes.

Being that this was a small and weakened kitten the low dose was sufficient.

A little cat vomited, suffered diarrhea, and did not eat. The little one was three months old. She already had experienced two visits to the vet and a number of shots with no signs of improvement.

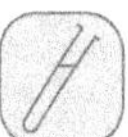

Treatment

First up I sought to find out by means of animal communication the reasons. The animal pointed out a woman that fed her things that did not become her. I proffered ½ drop of MMS in water directly in the mouth employing a syringe. Next day she received ½ drop three times. The diarrhea went away and with the first dose the little one began to eat again.

7.2.8 Epilepsy

Description practical example:

A young cat diagnosed with epilepsy came to the practice. First I ascertained the trigger for the illness using animal communication. Then I discussed further treatment with the owner.

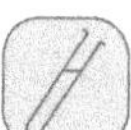

Treatment

We began with fine-tuned Schüssler Salts and dispensed 2 drops of activated MMS in approx.10 mL (0.338 fl oz) water 3 times daily. In three weeks the cat was doing better than she had in a long while, and that's how it stayed.

7.2.9 Cold

Description practical example:

The tomcat Carlo arrived for treatment suffering from a heavy cold with the following symptoms: Mucus ran from the eyes and nose, the ears were inflamed, he had watery diarrhea, and coughed and sneezed without end. He had trouble breathing.

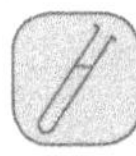

Treatment

MMS dosage: 2 drops of activated MMS in approx. 10 mL (0.338 fl oz) water. From this mix he received

approx. 3 mL (0.101 fl oz) once daily.

The number of drops of MMS and acid was increased by up to 4 drops of MMS and acid diluted with approx. 10 mL (0.338 fl oz) water of which he was given

approx. 3 mL (0.101 fl oz) directly in the mouth 1 time each day.

Thanks to MMS, changes to his diet, homeopathic medication suited to his needs, and inhalation, tomcat Carlo was healthy within one and a half weeks.

7.2.10 Feline immunodeficiency virus (FIV)

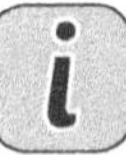

Feline immunodeficiency virus (FIV)

Feline immunodeficiency virus (FIV) is a virus belonging to the retroviridae family. The virus gives rise to an immunodeficiency sickness in cats (called cat aids colloquially) that closely resembles the human sickness AIDS.

Source: Wikipedia, last accessed May 28, 2015

Description practical example:

The cat of an acquaintance tested FIV positive. Fortunately the sickness had not yet broken out. Following this assessment the owner began administering MMS immediately.

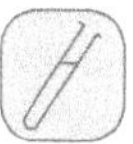

Day 1 - 2: 4 drops activated MMS with approx.10 mL (0.338 fl oz) water 2 times daily

Day 3 - 7: 6 drops activated MMS with approx.10 mL (0.338 fl oz) water 2 times daily

A pause of 3 days. Then 6 drops of activated MMS with approx.10 mL (0.338 fl oz) water were dispensed morning and evening for 1 week.

The treatment was a success. The sickness did not break out and the cat no longer tested positive.

7.2.11 Feline leukosis

Description practical example Elfie and Elroy:
"The kittens were born on a farm in Germany.

Unfortunately cat plague broke out there. Of the litter only a male and a female survived. They were very lucky for a German animal welfare worker rescued and kindly took them in. A great deal of time was spent on loving care by a cat-friendly married couple. Elfie and Elroy, as they were named, slowly recovered from their affliction.

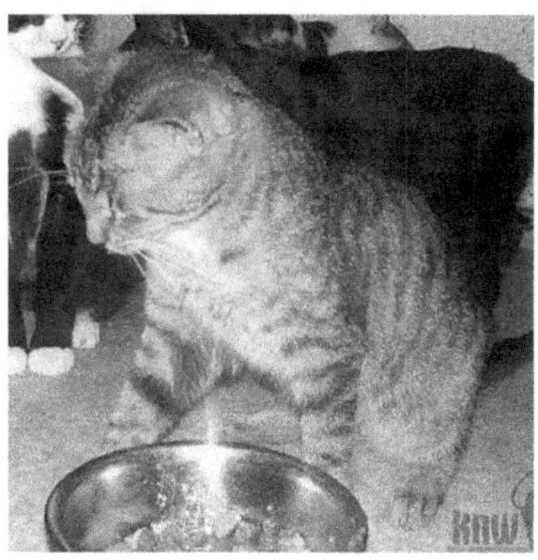

Elfie

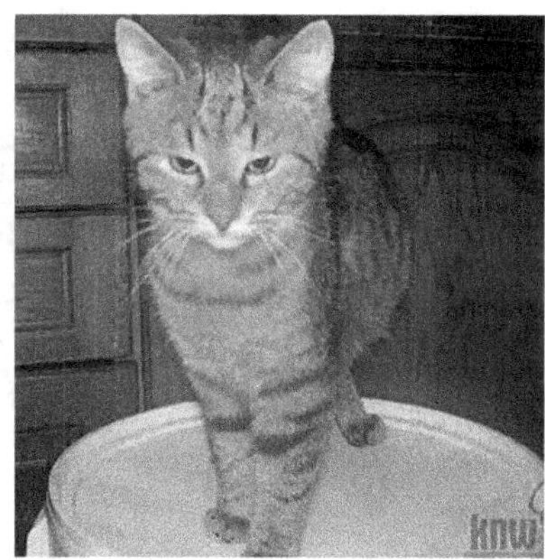

Elroy

The cat plague was overcome, but as so often happens the animal's suffering caused damage to the cerebellum and they were now afflicted by ataxia.

Elfie and Elroy were allowed to stay with the animal welfare couple and grew up with many pussyfoots. They were now about six months old.

Elfie's ataxia was relatively advanced and sometimes she toppled over when she was in a hurry. She did not understand how to use the cat litter tray and was still unclean.

Elroy was only slightly affected and the wobbly walk was only to be seen occasionally.

Despite their handicap they were spilling over with the joys of life. Elfie played and rampaged like a world champion as well.

But fate met the married couple full force: The Veterinary Office ordered them to disperse the whole troupe of cats. So began an urgent effort to find homes for them all; for Elfie and Elroy too.

The cuties were lucky for a second time, and rather than landing in an animal shelter they found a new home in Switzerland.

Elfie and Elroy were castrated beforehand.

Both had in the meantime settled in, they were healthy and it was delightful to see them radiating joy and energy. Elfie had even begun to use the litter tray.

Sadly, Elroy was diagnosed with feline leukosis."

We treated this so:

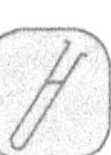

Treatment

More from the owner's report:

"My three-year-old tomcat Elroy would not eat for two day. On the third day I gave him MMS solution three times. This constituted 2 drops of MMS, acid activator and approx. 3 mL (0.101 fl oz) cream. In the evening he ate as usual.

I administered this dose for two weeks. On the afternoon of the first day we visited the vet where a blood sample was taken. The blood analysis indicated leukosis. That was two weeks ago. Since then he is again fit and eats normally. This was at the end of 2013. And now, almost two years on, Elroy is still doing fine."

7.2.12 Odor from the mouth

See: 7.1.23 "Dogs"

7.2.13 Skin infection, according to Veterinarian Dr. Schrader

Description practical example:
"Chlorine dioxide synthesized by us has long been employed with 100% success, especially for skin infections, and without causing any harm to patients.

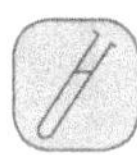

Treatment

For this purpose 20 drops of 22.5% sodium chlorite solution are mixed with 20 drops of 3.5% hydrochloric acid and dissolved in 60 mL (2.028 fl oz) cold tap water for exactly 1 minute. On account of the poisonous nature of the gases discharged production should take place under local exhaust ventilation, or alternatively, next to an open window.

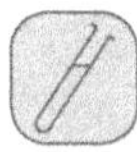

Continuation Treatment

Dabbing the infected regions of skin with this solution (a more intensive action takes place with prior treatment using 50% DMSO solution) results in the instantaneous elimination of all accessible microorganisms. For good measure the application should be repeated a number of times.
In cases of skin inflammation brought on by allergies, parallel treatment with cortisones and/or antihistamines is carried out at the same time."

7.2.14 Skin Problems

Description practical example:
The cat owner rang to explain that his cat had "acne" on its belly. That is how it appeared to him.

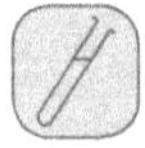

Treatment

As it was a very sweet cat he could dab the region twice a day with 8 drops of CDS and a little water. She was concurrently fed 8 drops of CDS with a little water and cream 2 times daily. After two weeks the skin problem was gone.

7.2.15 Cat head cold (rhinitis)

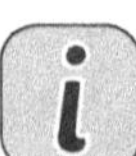

Disease of the upper respiratory passages

Phenotype: Sneezing, rhinitis, sniffles, conjunctivitis, agglutinated eyes and nostrils (with severe festering forms), fever

Causes: Caliciviruses, herpes viruses
This illness is common, especially with alley cats, particularly the young. Often the eyes weep to the extent of being purulent or glued up. The nose is in many cases also affected.

Description practical example 1:

A six-week-old kitten with a head cold was brought in to be treated. He suffered from diarrhea as well.

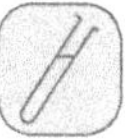

Treatment

A teaspoon of healing earth was administered mornings and evenings, plus an alternative medicine. The healing earth was stirred in with water and the mush produced was combined with the meal.

The head cold was treated with CDS. We began with 2 drops three times daily. Concurrently, the eyes were dabbed with a mixture of CDS and water. There was perceptible improvement, and then recovery.

Description practical example 2:

I live in a village and was given two kittens of about three weeks of age. Their noses were blocked and they had the sniffles, at times purulent.

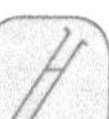

Treatment

I dispensed MMS in their food 3 times daily. I activated 1 drop of MMS, mixed it with 2 tablespoons of water, and gave each kitten half. One could see improvement with each day. Three months later they were bouncing around the house.

Description practical example 3:

This is not how it should turn out!

A baby kitten with a head cold was in a very poor state. It was an alley cat.

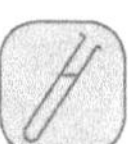

Treatment

We began the treatment with 2 drops of CDS 3 times daily, healing earth and Mumi-jo (See: Chapter 8.8). We dabbed the eyes with a CDS solution (12 drops CDS and

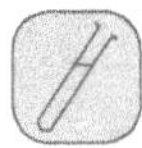

Continuation: Treatment

100 mL/3.381 fl oz water). The treatment brought improvement within a few days, but then the owner read an article about MMS in a newspaper, became uncertain, and went to a veterinarian. He administered the usual shot of antibiotics and whopped the little thing with a worm cure. From then on the kitten became weaker and weaker, dying after a few days.

If you are uncertain call a therapist or veterinarian who has worked with MMS or is open to it!

Of course it is not wise to speculate how it might have been … The press does have great influence though, as this example shows. Certainly, there may have been other reasons that caused the little cat to die. We can never know, regrettably.

7.2.16 Cancer

Description practical example:

The veterinarian confirmed a tumor under my cat's tongue. It was already very large and threatened to burst. My little one was consequently unable to eat and saliva dribbled from her mouth. Being that she was no longer young, having just turned nine, the vet thought that it might be best to put her down right away. I rejected this, and so he administered another shot of antibiotics and prescribed more of the same in tablet form. After two days her condition was deteriorating.

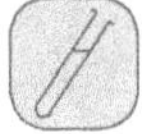

Treatment

I gave her 2 drops of activated MMS in water 2 times daily.
She allowed this to be squirted directly into the mouth with a syringe without complaint. After only two days her condition was improving. The tumor had vanished in two weeks.

7.2.17 Cancer in the oral cavity

Description practical example:

The 13 year-old tomcat Tommy - he came from an animal shelter - was in a very bad way ...

According to the veterinarian he had cancer in the oral cavity and thus required treatment with cortisone. Such medication would damage his kidneys even further (tests already indicated poor, almost not measurable, values).

Treatment

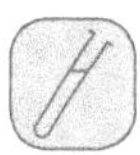

The treatment began with dietary changes, homeopathic medicine, and activated MMS (3 drops with 10 mL/0.338 fl oz water) of which 5 mL (0.169 fl oz) was provided 2 times daily. Tommy lived another two and half years.

7.2.18 Leucosis

Description practical example 1:

A tomcat diagnosed with leucosis arrived at the practice. He was emaciated; his fur was ragged and lusterless. The owner was verily worried about her darling for she had already lost two cats to leucosis.

Treatment

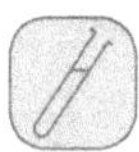

Firstly, we established the correct diet. In that he only ate fresh meat occasionally and was choosy regards high-grade canned food, nutrition was a constant challenge for the owner. He received, along with plant tinctures and homeopathic medicines, 8 drops of CDS in 10 mL (0.338 fl oz) water 3 times daily. This treatment lasted four weeks.

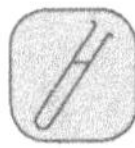

Continuation: Treatment

Today, almost two years on, the tom is healthy. His weight is normal and his fur lustrous.

Description practical example 2:

The patient was a stray tom in an awful state. He was emaciated, had a cold, and was listless. The veterinarian diagnosed leucosis and little hope of recovery. He advised the cat be put to sleep. I was not in agreement!

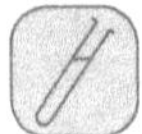

Treatment

I proceeded with a ten-day treatment as follows:

2 mL (0.067 fl oz) CDS solution (50 mL/1.690 fl oz water with 8 drops CDS) mornings and evenings for 2 days, 2 mL (0.067 fl oz) CDS solution hourly on the 3rd day.

His health improved daily.

7.2.19 Renal insufficiency (kidney failure)

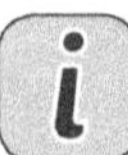

Kidney failure

The substances that ought be done away with were not sufficiently eliminated by the kidneys. Such failure can be acute, or advance slowly becoming chronic.

Phenotype: Attenuated urination, increasing urinary retention, and at a later stage vomiting, diarrhea, lack of appetite, significant water and electrolyte depletion

Causes: Shock and poisoning, incorrect nutriment

Emaciation and lusterless hair are often indications. A blood count should be done to clarify. Nutrition plays a major role with this malady. Dried food, which overtaxes the kidneys due to the long time it sits in the stomach on top of inadequate intake of liquid, is generally stipulated. This must be handled to suit each circumstance.

Description practical example 1:

A tomcat came to the practice diagnosed with renal failure.

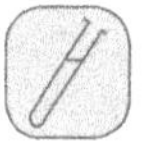

Treatment

I specified a special light diet to be provided, raw or lightly cooked. As an adjuvant he received homeopathic medicine. Three times a day 4 drops of CDS mixed with 10 mL (3.381 fl oz) water was administered directly into the mouth. After a week there was evident improvement. The fur was shiny and prettier, and the cat was more agile. Since then there have been no more problems with the kidneys. Food was switched to an exclusively BARF diet.

Description practical example 2:

A tomcat came to the practice diagnosed with renal failure.

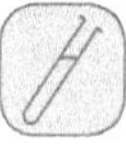

Treatment

He was given various Schüssler Salts and CDS. The switch to raw meat was implemented here as well.

For 1 week he was given 4 drops of CDS with 10 mL (0.338 fl oz) water 3 times daily.

Three weeks later his blood values were tested. The indications were normal, and six months later the blood values were excellent.

7.2.20 Kidney problems

Description practical example:

A twelve-year-old cat with kidney problems came to the practice.
He was skeletal, and his fur dull. In spite of his age we sought to

switch him over to a higher standard of nutrition. He was very picky though, and what he would eat this week he would not look at the next. This was for the owner a real challenge.

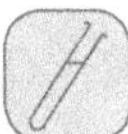

Treatment

The tom was dispensed homeopathic medications, Terrakraft extract, and 8 drops of CDS in 10 mL (0.338 fl oz) water 3 times daily for 10 days.

The situation was acute and so the tom received the full dose from the beginning; he tolerated this well. This is definitely not doable with every cat! Two years have passed and he is doing very well indeed. He has put on weight, his fur shines, and it is still suspense packed finding food that the "Sir" will accept.

7.2.21 Parvovirus and allergies

Description practical example:

The cat rescue center reached me with the following concerned message:

"Accompanying I send some photos of little Mickey. Mickey's mama was relocated to a new home yesterday. Mickey, with her scratch guard around her neck, was for the mama a little suspect, and she mostly ran away. Mickey purrs as soon as she is touched, is very disposed towards humans. Together with her mama Babsi I adopted her from an allotment garden settlement at the beginning of October. Brother Moritz and sister Maxi died of parvovirus.

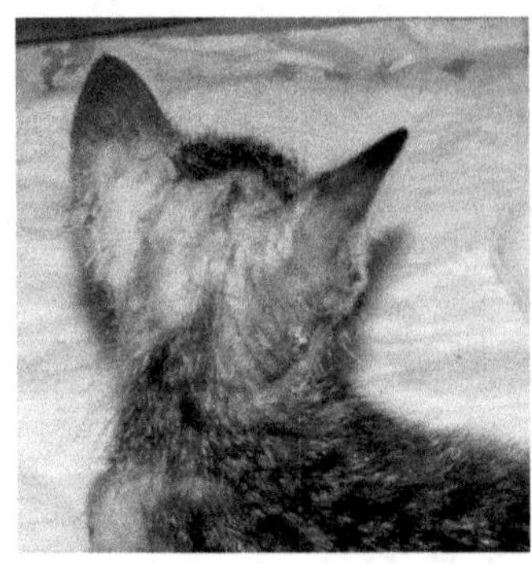
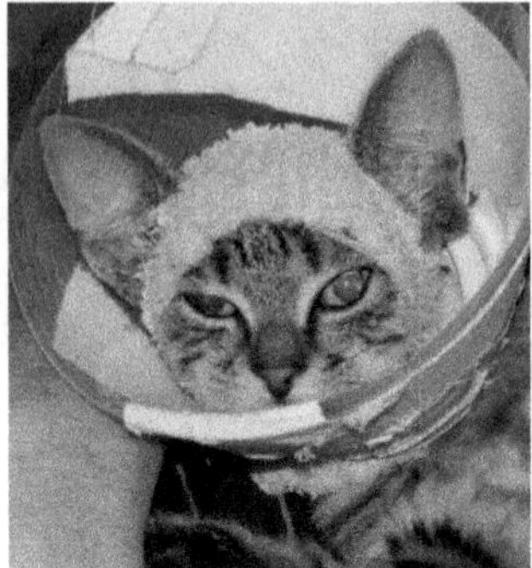

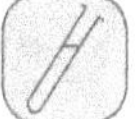

Treatment

The treatment went like this:

We dispensed 6 drops of MMS/DMSO in 100 mL (0.338 fl oz) water. In addition a narrow-leafed plantain marigold salve was prescribed, plus a plant tincture called Seelenfreude (soul joy). To follow the discontinuation of cortisone salve and the recommended treatment there was immediate and resounding success. Mickey would not drink the MMS. We took off her collar and spread a great deal of the solution over the whole body, especially the front legs. Mickey licked this off carefully, so taking in the MMS orally. It worked.

Here are pictures of Mickey after three weeks!
We dabbed MMS lotion onto a hematoma that the foster mother noticed during the treatment, it faded completely. All in all the cat is making real progress!"

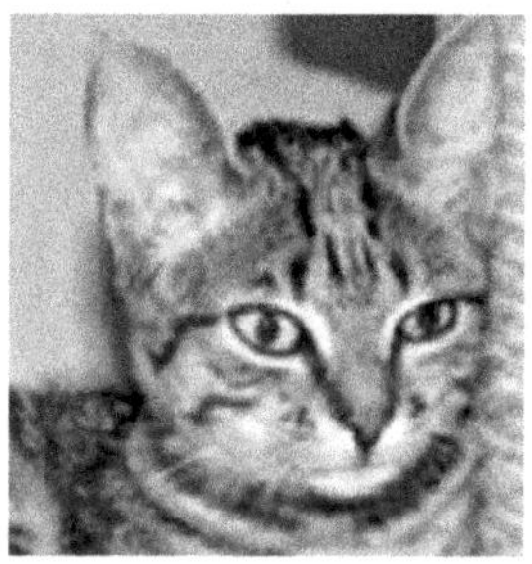
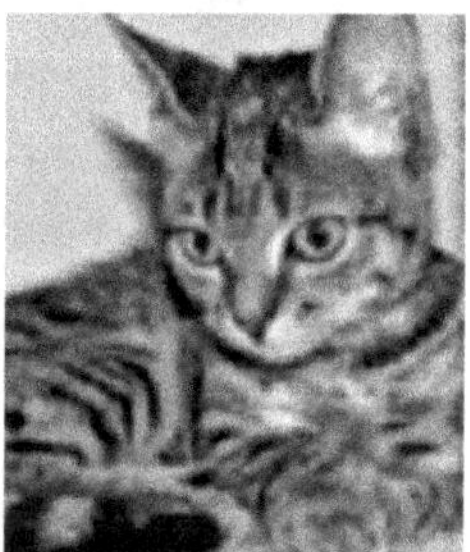

7.2.22 Fungus

Description practical example:
A nineteen-year-old cat had a fungus and almost no fur on this spot.

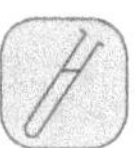

Treatment

The owner rubbed in activated MMS diluted in water (unfortunately the amounts are not documented) on the area a number of times daily. After a few days the fungus was gone.

7.2.23 Piddles in the apartment

Description practical example:

Brought in for treatment was a cat, three years old and castrated, that piddles all over the apartment. In the opinion of the veterinarian it was all clear-cut. Even a bladder puncture was carried out, without results. His assessment was that she was basically healthy.

By means of animal communication she showed me that she longed to go outside.

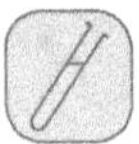

Treatment

She was given Schüssler Salts and a Bach flower; naturally the cat was now allowed to go outside! After a few days an improvement was discernible, though time and again there were setbacks.

After some time she received 8 drops of CDS in 10 mL (0.338 fl oz) water 3 times daily plus a common daisy tincture: Look and see! Within a week the problem had vanished. Here too, it was unnecessary to increase the dosage slowly, but she tolerated the medications without difficulties.

Take care with a bladder puncture! Bacteria can flourish in the bladder and thus set off further major problems.

7.2.24 Streptococci

Description practical example:

I had a tomcat with streptococci as a patient in the practice.

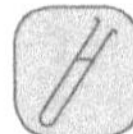

Treatment

I treated the tom with 4 - 5 drops of Gefeu (with water) 3 times daily direct in the mouth. The problem was soon resolved.

7.2.25 Toxoplasmosis

Description practical example:

A fourteen-year-old cat, truly a Madame, was brought to me suffering toxoplasmosis. According to the veterinarian she indicated a value of over 300, which is very high. Antibiotics were administered, but there was no improvement.

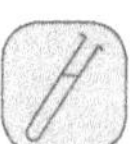

Treatment

On the first day we tried an hourly dose of 8 drops CDS to which she responded after only a few measures by vomiting. As she resisted medicament of all kinds and accepted no treats we were forced to be resourceful. The only way to treat this cat was to put the medicine on her paw, which she then licked clean. So we gave her 1 drop of CDS on the paw 3 - 5 times daily. She tolerated this small amount and accepted it readily. She received 2 drops of lady's thistle tincture the same way. Evenings, she was given a pinch of zeolite in water mixed in with her meal. To increase her physical strength she was given Spirulina and a soupçon of Reishi mushroom.

With every day there was improvement. The cat visibly found joy in life. Her condition has been stable for a year.

7.2.26 Unknown problem

Description practical example:

A stray approached our house circumspectly. Its fur lacked luster and was ragged. When I was able to briefly touch him I felt thick ropes like with a heavily pregnant female.

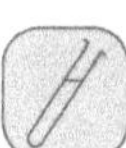

Treatment

The tom was very shy, so I mixed 2 drops of activated MMS in water with his food mornings and evenings. A couple of days later I spotted him defecating

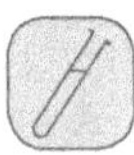

Continuation: Treatment

near the house. What I then saw was a shock. It was excrement mixed with a great deal of yellow plastic. From that moment on there was a real upturn. He received 2 drops of MMS in his food for some time. The fur began to shine and the tom developed gloriously. He has been living with us for around two years, though he is only slowly becoming hand-tame. He has had a skin problem during this time with scurf and crust on his back. I gave him 6 drops of activated MMS diluted in water for this. I drew some into a syringe and slowly distributed the contents under the fur (no needle, and not under the skin) and carefully massaged it in. This he enjoyed. As he always cleaned himself, a small amount of the drops was ingested as well. Following just a few applications it was hardly there to see.[1]

---

[1] I would like to comment further on the case portrayed. It of course makes more sense and is more effective to administer MMS separately to food. In practice my experience is, especially with cats, that to dispense the medicine can often be tricky and that our cuddly cats transmute into guerrilla fighters.

In such situations the attitude of the owner plays a central role. Am I disgusted in the course of the preparation? Have I doubts that my animal will accept the medicine? Our animal senses these feelings, is instantly aware "whoopsy-daisy, something is not ok here!" and then all too often it s no go.

It is likely that various dosages occur to you. But of course every animal responds differently to MMS just as it does to other medications. I attempt to attune myself to the animal concerned. I do this by means of animal communication (See: chapter 14). During the first conversation with the owner I often sense that the animal is very sensitive. In such a case I cannot begin with a high dose, the animal would promptly vomit or suffer diarrhea. Given that often the animal is already weakened by the disorder it would be counterproductive for the treatment, might even be a retrograde step.

7.2.27 Digestion problems

Description practical example:

A friend called. Her somewhat overweight cat had digestion problems. Up front: Both cat and owner are fastidious.

Treatment 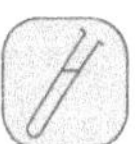

I advised: 2 drops of activated MMS thinned with water administered with a syringe directly into the mouth. There was great skepticism. So what came to pass? The cat accepted this without a song and dance, and on the second day even begged while the drops were being prepared. This was certainly a lesson learned for the owner. The problem with digestion was already a thing of the past on the second day.

7.2.28 Tooth inflammation

Description practical example:

A cat came to the practice with inflamed gums. The veterinarian wanted to pull the teeth right away. The cat had strong bad breath as well; the blood values were poor due to the inflammation. The owner was very fearful, so we set forth with extreme care.

Treatment 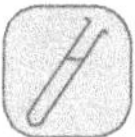

½ drop MMS in approx. 5 mL (0.169 fl oz) water 3 times daily for 2 days;
1 drop MMS in approx. 5 mL (0.169 fl oz) water 3 times daily for 2 days;
2 drops MMS in approx. 5 mL (0.169 fl oz) water 3 times daily.

At the end of the week an improvement was to be seen. The bad breath was hardly discernible. But for a pinhead-size point the inflammation had shrunken. We continued the treatment in this way: Mix 4 drops of CDS with water in a shot glass, dab the mix onto the wound with a cotton swab many times in the day.

Concurrently, we changed over to a light, raw meat diet. A year later she still had all her teeth, no inflammation, and no halitosis. She was very well.

7.3 Equine disorders that have been successfully treated with MMS

7.3.1 Abscess

Description practical example:

I treated an abscess directly on the saddle girth (a tick? a sting?) of my Wallach with MMS spray + 40% DMSO and coated the wound with honey (as with my seniors). The wound opened up and could then be expressed. Subsequently, I again applied MMS spray and honey until epithelization was complete (four days). Everything is now healed and looks wonderful. Unfortunately I did not write down the dosages.

7.3.2 Breathing problem

Description practical example:

"Fantasy girl began to cough slightly in March.

In April she was coughing up sputum, light yellow and stringy, especially when bearing weight. She was given large amounts of homeopathic agents, and the therapies that for me were standard up to that point in time. This had all proved to be ineffective by June.

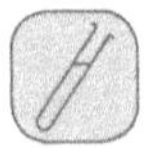

Treatment

Beginning in July I dispensed MMS 3 times daily.

Inside a week the dosage increased from 10 drops MMS with 200 mL (6.763 fl oz) water to 200 drops MMS (10 mL/0.338 fl oz) and 400 mL (13.525 fl oz) water.

The rasping cough, which was very stubborn, subsided appreciably after three weeks. By September she expectorated only occasionally. There were days of absolutely no coughing and others when she coughed lightly. We were very pleased for there was progress.

By the end of September she had more air volume and only a little runny slime, following physical activity mostly, and the irritation of the throat had all but disappeared.

To be completely rid of the problem we have begun inhalations of sole.

As an adjunct we have provided the first sole mist inhalation:

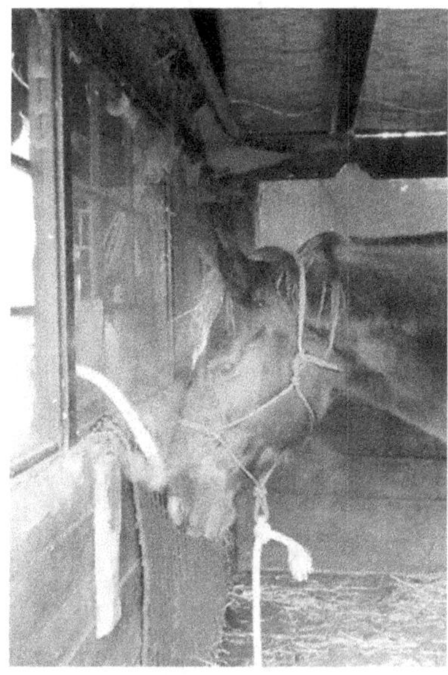

In the beginning: no discharge.

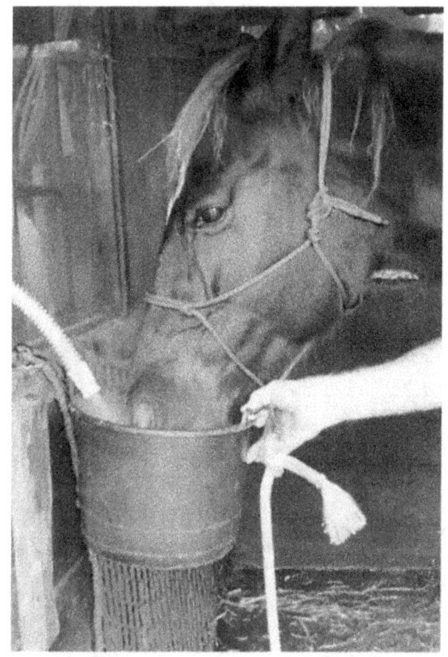

After 15 minutes the discharge occurred by itself as we rode at a tilt and a gentle gallop through the forest for 30 minutes.

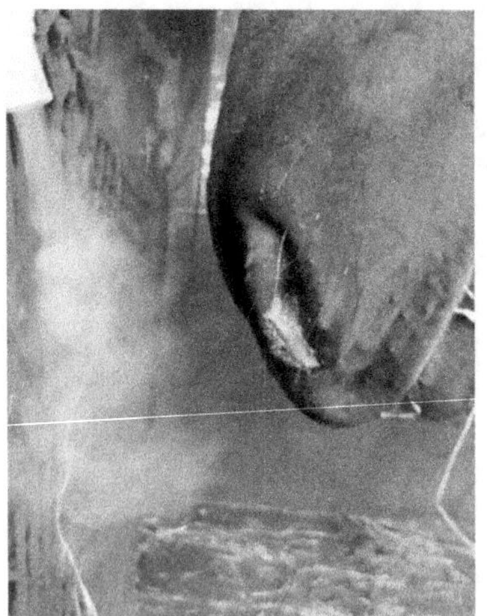 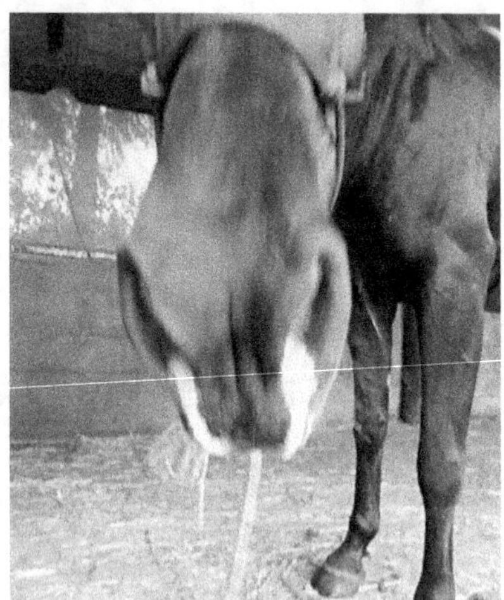

The discharge recurred after riding, but it was noticeably more liquid than in July and August.

Here we can see how the nasal mucus loosened, and ran out freely. Thanks to MMS we had already gotten rid of the cough."

7.3.3 Eye inflammation

Description practical example:
Our mare had been going to the veterinarian for more than three years due to an inflammation of the eye. The vet could provide neither the grounds nor a diagnosis, but administered antibiotics repeatedly, salves et cetera -this was of course costly. Despite the treatment the eye was very swollen and the mare suffered a perpetual flood of tears. When one touched the area carefully it was very hot.

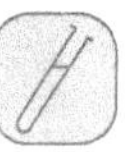

Treatment

I performed the internal treatment like this:

Day 1: 10 drops MMS with approx. 200 mL (6.762 fl oz) apple puree 3 times daily.
Day 2: 20 drops MMS with approx. 300 mL (10.144 fl oz) apple puree 3 times daily.

The swelling went down and the eye became clearer as soon as day 2. I dispensed 20 drops mornings and evenings for another 2 weeks - there were no more signs of inflammation. To this day there has been no reoccurrence.

7.3.4 Cushing syndrome

Description practical example,
after a report by Michaela von Jähnichen:

"Rosi, a Haflinger mare born 19.05.1996, became ill with the metabolic disorder of Cushing approximately two years ago.

Despite Pergolide, focussed dietary changes and other treatments she hardly improved. She did not want to leave her stall, there was always the suspicion that she suffered laminitis."

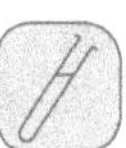

Treatment

"I learned of MMS through a telephone consultation with the veterinary practice of Michaela von Jähnichen. In that it was probably the last chance for my horse I began the treatment despite great misgivings on 18.04.2014.

Initially I gave her 10 drops in the morning on an empty stomach to which she responded a little later by lying down in her stall. I did not know if this was due to the drops, therefore I reduced the count to 8 drops twice daily after speaking with Michaela on the second day.

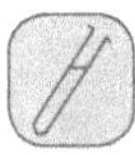

Continuation: Treatment

On the third day we increased the dose to 10 drops. Now we waited until she had eaten some hay - we wanted to ensure that she did not get queasy again. On the fourth day we increased the dosage to 3 times 12 drops. My horse improved daily, and I became more confident each day.

The fifth day Rosi wanted to be with the other horses in the enclosure again. I gave her 15 drops 3 times. On the sixth day I mixed in DMSO as a booster. The following days I increased the dosage to 15 drops mixed with carrot or apple juice, 4 times.

Next I called a break, but then when Rosi was again unwell I gave her MMS immediately. An additional tip from Frau von Jähnichen was the Lifewave patch. On days when the hooves caused difficulties I attached Lifewave patches to all four hooves.

Something that became evident to us at the end of two months was that the subcutaneous fat under the crest had decreased and that the hardened musculature on the neck was suppler. We assumed that on days that Rosi walked poorly that the body was decontaminating due to the MMS, as on previous days she had been fine and even galloped with the herd."

7.3.5 EORTH - painful tooth disease

Description practical example,
report from Monika Lehmkühler:

"At the beginning of 2011 (21. 02. 2011) a permanent gingival inflammation was discovered in Uno's mouth. We headed off to the horse dentist. X-rays were made and the diagnosis was Equine Odontoclastic Tooth Resorption and Hypercementosis (EOTRH).

Uno's illness was in the initial stages, but nonetheless considered incurable.

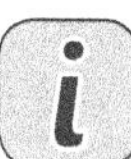

EORTH

This condition that usually affects the incisors can only be stopped by adding a vital mushroom to the feed. Horses exhibit varying indications of discomfort or pain. Mostly horses of more than fifteen years of age are affected.

Uno turned fifteen in April 2011.

First of all, the diagnosis was a shock. In the Internet we found, almost exclusively, reports discussing teeth being pulled and horses that suffered extreme pain.

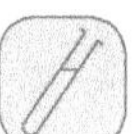

Treatment

Since then we have used Equident Oral Care (vital mushrooms) every day: 1.5 measuring spoons daily in the beginning - in the meantime we have reduced this to a ½ measuring spoon daily - mixed in with his beet slices.

In April 2011 his general condition was poor (no growth in the hooves, and, most obviously, dull fur). Consequently we arranged for a blood count: Iron and zinc values were noticeably low. We have fed him Atcom Huf Vital ever since, his condition has thus improved.

In June 2011 we visited the horse dentist once more. The EORTH was slightly worse. We received an antibiotic of which we sprayed 10 mL (0.338 fl oz) directly into Uno's mouth daily. Every two days the teeth and gums were rubbed with Chlorhexidine.

In August 2011 we changed the bridle over from a bitless bridle to a LG bridle from Monika Lehmenkühler; we heard of MMS there. Since August 2011 Uno has been administered MMS as follows:

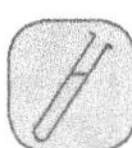

Continuation: Treatment

05.08.2011: Began with 1 x 10 drops MMS orally + apple puree every day; increased every second day by 5 drops until 7 days later (14.08.2011) 1 x 30 drops was attained.

14.08.2011 - 04.09.2011: Daily 1 x 30 drops MMS + apple puree.

Pause

30.09.2011: Resumed slowly with 1 x 10 drops increasing to reach 1 x 30 drops by 09.10.2011.

09.10. - 08.11.2011: 1 x 30 drops MMS + apple pure daily.

Pause: Clean teeth daily with 4 drops MMS in a little water.

November 2011: New X-ray at the dentist. EOTRH has not worsened. The condition of the teeth has not changed. Uno's teeth were shortened with every visit.

We reduced the Vital mushrooms to 1 measuring spoon daily; Equident reduced from 08.12.2011 to 0.5 measuring spoons daily.

Between 09. - 17.12. 2011: MMS increased from 1 to 31 drops.

Between 19.12. - 19.01.2012: 1 x 31 drops MMS + apple puree.

Pause: 20. 01. - 20.02.2012

Between 21.02. - 01.03.2012 MMS increased from 1 x 10 to 31 drops daily.

Pause

Between 28.05. - 06.06.2012 MMS increased from 1 x 10 to 31 drops daily.

Between 07.08. - 09.08.2012 MMS increased from 1 x 10 to 31 drops daily.

Between 10.08. - 05.09.2012 1 x 31 drops MMS daily.

Pause

Between 05.10. - 07.10.2012 MMS increased from 1 x 10 to 31 drops daily.

An X-ray made in October 2012 indicated improvement. On one side of the tooth the swelling brought on by EOTRH had vanished (See: X-ray image)."

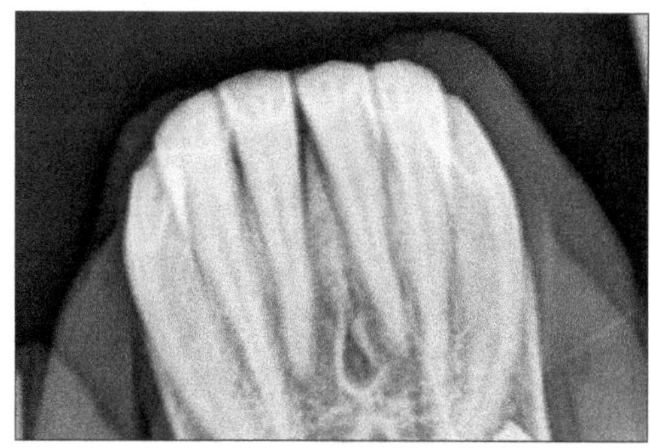

7.3.6 Grass mites

Description practical example:
A horse suffered grass mites.

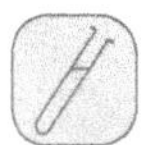

Treatment

It was washed 2 times daily with MMS: a 10 L (2.641 gal) bucket containing 5 L (1.320 gal) of water mixed with 20 drops of activated MMS. There was definite improvement after only 2 days.

After a successful treatment it is important to follow up with homeopathy - to memorize, so to say, the success.

The horse was given the following dose of MMS orally: To begin 40 drops of MMS increasing to 120 drops diluted in 400 mL (13.525 fl oz) water. At the same time the feed was adjusted and the metabolism activated. It was a slow process, but there was continual improvement.

With horses as well it is important to ask: What are they fed? It is especially important to check the constituents of the pre-prepared mixes on offer. It can do no harm to read the ingredients list and to occasionally ask questions. Not all that is on offer and considered to be normal is good.

7.3.7 Grass mites, itching

Description practical example:

Here is a tale about our pony Blitz. It all began with small bites that began to ooze. Apparently it itched intensely and the pony constantly rubbed himself against the gate of his stall. In he beginning the area was the size of the head of a thumbtack, but it grew large due to the rubbing. I continually rinsed it and disinfected, and applied salve; nothing helped though.

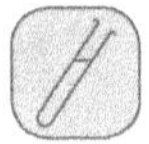

Treatment

I applied MMS, 10 drops in water mixed in with the feed, twice daily, and washed the wound with MMS one or two times a day. In a glass bowl I mixed 10 drops of activated MMS and mixed this with water. I then folded a paper towel to about the size of the wound and dunked this in the bowl. I now placed the wet paper towel on the spot and allowed it to soak in for around five minutes. I then attempted to remove the crust.

After another five minutes I laid on a cloth soaked in MMS - done! This treatment continued for four days (See photographs). I administered MMS for roughly a week in total. The final picture shows how the fur was growing again. All is well now.

By the by: Six weeks later, Namira, our South German Coldblood mare, was affected by the same problem as Blitz. I began treating her with MMS without delay and at the end of a week it was all cleared up (I used the right methods from the start ...).

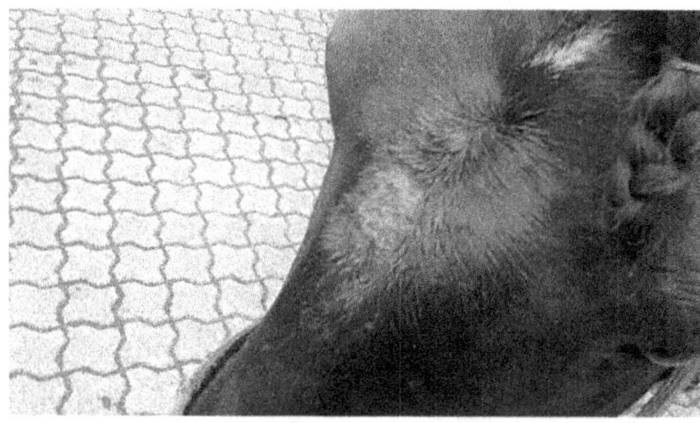

prior to treatment

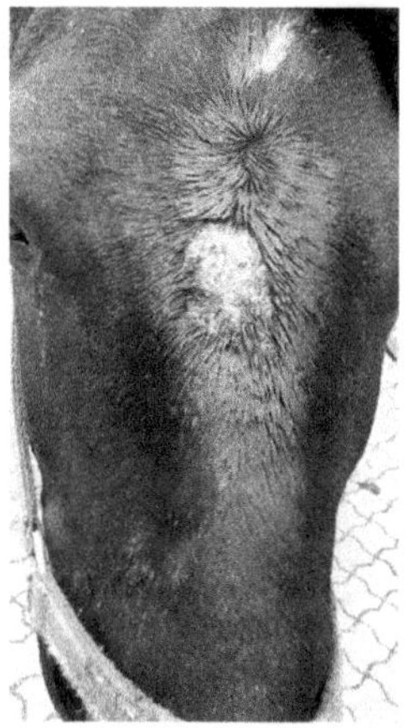

following the initial treatment

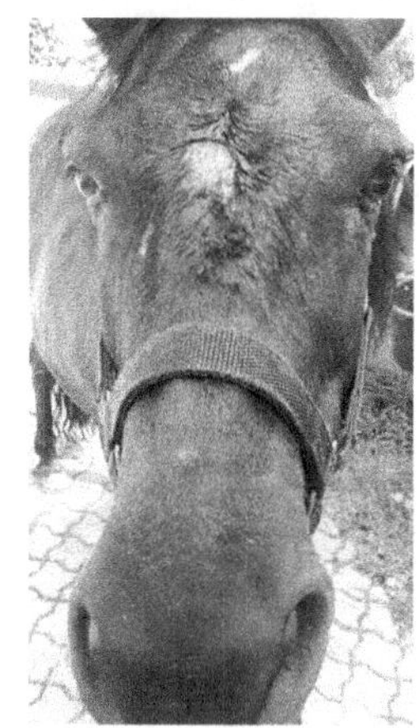

after four days

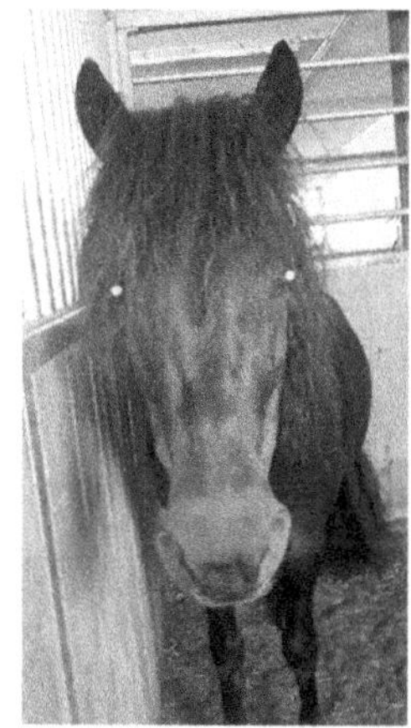

following three or four weeks

7.3.8 Hoof cancer

Protocol of the treatment of a horse suffering hoof cancer with MMS

Description practical example, report by Veronika W.:

"A Wallach, now three years old, in his first winter suffered as a foal from persistent thrush in the front left hoof - this was treated conservatively (cleaning, scraping, commercial hoof spray et cetera).

When about two and a half years of age the horse was stalled and the thrush treated more intensively (still using conservative methods), albeit without success.

In July 2010 the condition worsened. The thrush increasingly developed according to the classic mold into hoof cancer: Softening of the whole horny layer; slimy, cheesy film, et cetera.

The consulting specialist diagnosed hoof cancer.

Mid July 2010 the horse was treated locally with a salve[1] that seemed promising at first: To the eye, there was rapid improvement - the hoof became horny again.

Unfortunately the next appointment at the blacksmith revealed that the effect was only on the outer layer, the hoof cancer was still present deeper in.

We broke off with the salve and settled on surgery.

The appointment was to be October 1, 2010.

---

1 **Note regarding the salve:** The mixture is highly poisonous, and due to the prohibited ingredient Phenol is difficult to obtain. Hence, we had the salve mixed abroad. We consider the salve to be effective so long as the persistent condition can be defined as thrush and has not advanced to the stage of being hoof cancer.

Here is the formula:
75 g/2.645 oz zinc oxide
75 g/2.645 oz copper acetate
2.5 g/0.088 oz fluorouracil
20 g/0.705 oz liquid phenol
90 g/3.174 oz liquid paraffin
500 g/17.636 oz yellow Vaseline as carrier

Author's comment: This is not the black salve.

The cancer-like material was thoroughly removed from deep inside the hoof tissue under general anesthetic. A chicken-egg-size hole, had to be closed by means of a metal cap with an internal compression dressing.

This was an enormous strain on the horse as it was necessary to replace the dressing daily, at first under sedation, and then every two or three days. The animal was an in-patient at the clinic.

Subsequent to the operation progress was at first good. The hoof slowly healed deep into its center.

In November 2010 the physician in charge informed us that despite the ongoing treatment the hoof was again cancerous. A new operation was ruled out.

Seeing that there were no alternatives to the treatment implemented it was suggested we seriously consider putting the horse to sleep if there were no new developments regarding the illness within the next couple of weeks.

We heard of MMS for the first time at this point, and despite a lack of information in the literature regarding hoof cancer we decided spontaneously to treat the horse with MMS.

The horse was given MMS orally. The regime is supplied below. The affected hoof was locally disinfected with a MMS solution in addition: twice daily to begin, then daily after a few days, and later each time a fresh dressing was applied (i.e., two to three times in the week).

The horse was locally treated with Novaderma in parallel. This salve was administered each time the bandage was changed and left on until the next change of dressing.

The first course of treatment with MMS lasted approximately three weeks. At the end of three days the cancer had retreated appreciably; a few days more and the cancer was no longer perceivable. We then took a break of about two weeks, and thereafter we repeated the course with MMS.

The MMS protocol:

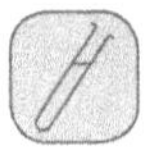

Treatment

We began with 15 drops MMS + activator, mornings and evenings daily.

Seeing as the horse exhibited no signs of discomfort and never suffered diarrhea, the dose was increased by 5 drops each day until 100 drops of MMS mornings and evenings was reached. The amount of water was also increased from 100 mL (3.381 fl oz) to 1 L (33.814 fl oz: this is very important as 100 drops of activated MMS is very caustic and is therefore dangerous.

To begin the activated MMS was mixed with apple juice and squirted directly into the horse's mouth. Later we simply stirred the MMS (mixed with a half glass of apple juice) in with the concentrated feed. The horse was not impressed, but emptied the trough anyway. Only at the end stages were we obliged to employ tricks such as mixing in apple slices, treats, and so on.

The horse is today, a good year on from the first diagnosis, free of hoof cancer, and enjoys the best of health.

Owing to the operation the hoof is appreciably retracted, and in the region where the disease was there is a deep cleft remaining. The condition continues to improve and we hope that as far as is possible the hoof has within a year reverted to the usual form.

Otherwise the hoof grows quite normally. The horse walks bare-hooved, was in fact never lame, and is worked as usual.

We are convinced that MMS rescued this horse filled with life's promise, and this without side effects despite the high doses!

Some notes on the side:
January 6, 2011 we brought the horse home, some three months after the operation. It had stood in the stall for a good three months, mostly so it would not wound itself with the heavy metal cap.

The horse was despite the extended history of sickness astoundingly fit, and had a great need to move due to the long period of standing. We decided to leave the Wallach in the paddock in spite of the iron cap.

To this purpose we padded and heavily taped the complete hoof including the iron cap. Even with this brick on his leg he moved normally in no time at all, and along with his female companion raced to and fro.

Towards the beginning of February the hoof had grown back in the center to the extent that the dermis was coated with a thin, horny coating. We removed the iron cap while retaining the sticking-tape bandage for a couple more weeks. Early March the bandaging was discontinued and the horse was once again saddled up.

The requisite almost daily renewal of the outside bandage was of course tedious, but we believe that the approach to husbandry plays a major role in an effective convalescence.
Our opinion is that young horses and small children belong outside in the open air.

In conclusion, our advice to all those who have a horse standing in the stall suffering from persistent thrush, especially when the husbandry conditions are good, and it is a question of only one hoof while the other hooves are free of thrush:

Don t take this lightly!

We are convinced that we could have spared the horse a long and painful road, and ourselves a good five-figure sum, if we had of done something concrete and at an early juncture about the thrush - like a systematic local treatment with MMS, the salve described above, or the easy to come by Nova-derm salve that any veterinarian can provide.

MMS is after all probably not only the best, but the cheapest choice as well!

Meanwhile, the horse is now seven years old, is healthy and performs successfully at L-Dressage.

7.3.9 Laminitis

Description practical example:
"My horse is light, weighs approximately 500 kg (1102.312 lb).

Treatment

I began with 15 drops of MMS + activator + approx. 200 mL (06.762 fl oz) water orally, for two days, then I increased to 20 drops 2 times daily.

If no diarrhea occurred, the next day I went up to 30 drops 2 times daily, then 35 drops 2 times daily and then stayed with this dosage. We could have given the horse a high dose of up to 50 drops without problems. After two weeks we reduced to 1 measure each day for five weeks.

After that my horse completely recovered from his laminitis.

The illness never returned.

My Wallach receives MMS 2 to 3 times yearly for colds and cough besides - that suffices.

We have had our peace for years now!"

7.3.10 Laminitis due to Poisoning

Description practical example:

I attended to a seven-year-old mare with a serious case of laminitis due to poisoning. Hitherto, a veterinarian had treated her with antibiotics bringing no improvement. She lay down for most of the day afterwards and had therefore developed lesions.

As there was no improvement at all after two more weeks we set about treating her with MMS and DMSO. Her musculature overall had stiffened considerably, so she received a homeopathic medicine in addition.

Treatment
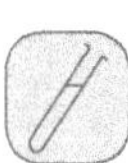

Dosage (oral):

Day 1: 10 drops MMS + 1 mL (0.033 fl oz/approx. 20 drops) DMSO + approx. 200 mL (6.762 fl oz) water

Day 2: 20 drops MMS + 1 mL (0.033 fl oz/approx. 20 drops) DMSO + approx. 300 mL (10.144 fl oz) water

Day 3: 30 drops MMS + 2 mL (0.067 fl oz /approx. 40 drops) DMSO + approx. 400 mL (13.525 fl oz) water

Day 4: 40 drops MMS + 2 mL (0.067 fl oz /approx. 40 drops) DMSO + approx. 400 mL (13.525 fl oz) water

She was longed daily in order to stimulate her humors as well. On the second day she was already somewhat better.

Following a break she was given 40 drops 2 times daily over two weeks.

The raw patches on the body healed, and now she is walking almost normally.

7.3.11 Lip torn-off

Description practical example, report by Eva H.:
"I stabled my horse. Unfortunately the horse was left in the stall wearing her head-collar in spite of my instructions to always remove it. This Sunday, while at home, I had a strange feeling. I said to my husband: 'We must go to the stables!' and immediately the phone rang, something was not right with my mare! I drove there and my heart fell: The whole upper lip was hanging by only a thread. I immediately rang my veterinarian. He said he could do nothing; I ought go to the animal clinic.

During the drive to the stables a name floated around my head, a veterinarian who I had not met, though his wife had come to me for pain therapy. I called the untried veterinarian - he came without delay.

Meanwhile I took care of my mare. First I had to collect all the good, positive energy inside of me, then I entered her box, began to comb her down and said: 'You are the most beautiful and the best,' and so on. This I could only do through my positive energy. In that moment I did not suffer along with her, but imparted something positive and uplifting (difficult to describe).

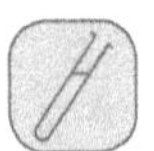

Treatment

The veterinarian was amazed on arriving to find a fearless, even-tempered horse. He was obliged to completely separate the upper lip. The mare was given homeopathic medicine - the vet being very unorthodox he allowed me to administer it. The mare was not given antibiotics, but CDS in her drinking trough instead:
40 drops twice daily plus 20 drops of DMSO.

Furthermore: There were many voices insisting that I put the horse down. I had to contend with massive hostility.

Nonetheless the horse fed on its hay and concentrated food. It had to develop a new eating technique. At no point did it suffer fever or pain!"[1]

7.3.12 Pastern Dermatitis/Mud fever with foals

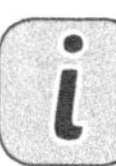

What is Pastern Dermatitis?

Pastern dermatitis is a bacterial skin inflammation in the hoof bulb that mostly affects horses with long hair in the pastern region. This disease occurs mostly in the winter months. Causes include stabling, hygiene, long hair in the pastern region, and the grass in autumn.

Description practical example 1,
report by Cornelia S.:

I used MMS successfully against mud fever.
It was a Tinker foal with long hair.

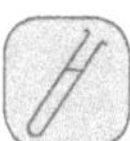

Treatment

"We mixed 10 drops of MMS + activator with 100 mL (3.381 fl oz) water and sprayed the affected regions 2 times daily. After about two weeks the pastern dermatitis had vanished."

---

1   "I always use CDS in the stall or with animals, as it is easier to handle. MMS would be just as good, though in smaller doses. Please consult an experienced person you trust or a specialist."

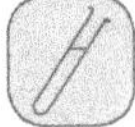

Description practical example 2, report by Cornelia S.::

The hind legs of our horse were visibly swollen as well. I applied MMS without delay.

Treatment

"I dribbled 50 drops of activated MMS in a bucket which I then filled to half. I washed the legs with this. In the evening I wrapped a cloth soaked in the same solution around the legs, and covered this with plastic bags fixed with bandage. Already by the next day the swelling was less.

I dispensed 80 drops of activated MMS mixed with water and wheat bran orally 3 times a day. This mix was proffered for two weeks, the legs washed, and the crust cleaned every couple of days."

7.3.13 Penis swollen

Description practical example, report by Ursula W.:

A thirteen-year-old Wallach's penis was so swollen he could hardly walk.

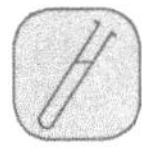

Treatment

"First I applied quark to cool, because quark draws toxins. The Wallach did not like this at all and the effect was insufficient. I then sprayed MMS solution onto it 3 times daily; the penis recovered somewhat, his temperature was 39.6 °C (103.28 °F). I gave then him 14 drops of MMS with 200 mL (06.762 fl oz) water and 5 mL (0.169 fl oz/ approx. 100 drops) of 60% DMSO 2 times daily. After a day my Wallach moved more easily and ate normally again. Nevertheless, I called in the veterinarian, who applied an infusion with 14 drops of MMS and 5 mL (0.169 fl oz/approx. 100 drops) of DMSO. The penis had detumesced on the left, on the right it was still a little swollen. I then engaged an animal natural health practitioner who determined

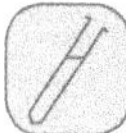

Continuation: Treatment

that the left side was fine the blood being red. On the right side the blood was almost black indicating blood poisoning. My Wallach received 9 drops of MMS with dextrogyral lactic acid and 200 mL (06.762 fl oz) water 1 time each day for a week, plus 10 drops of propolis drops 1 time daily, and 1 Artemesia capsule. He is not yet in top form, but is on the way. The trigger was presumably a tick bite on the penis."

7.3.14 Blow to the Shoulder

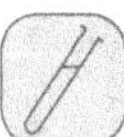

Treatment (report by Ursula W.)

"A blow to the right shoulder of a mare was treated with MMS spray and 50% DMSO spray for three days. (A recipe for a MMS spray is to be found in Chapter 6.3.3) The mare did not go lame for a single day and the shoulder was not sensitive to the touch."

7.3.15 Summer Eczema

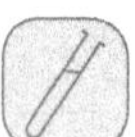

Treatment Tip

This "problem" occurs frequently in summer. It is helps greatly to wash with water fortified with MMS with the first signs. I strongly encourage the stimulation of the metabolism. This must correspond to the needs of each individual horse. It is equally important to track down the cause of the problem. Mostly a response comes too late, and then to save the situation aggressive substances are employed. One more aspect should be taken into account: Most horse keepers proceed as though the eczema will reappear each year. This must not be.

7.3.16 Injury to the Leg

Description practical example:

A horse was injured on the hind leg; exhibited a cut running laterally.

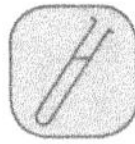

Treatment

Approximately 10 drops of 50% DMSO was applied, and then 10 drops of CDS spread on top. There were no outgrowths, everything healed perfectly.

7.3.17 Warts

Description practical example, report by Karin R.

A horse came to be treated for a pervasive attack of warts. There had been many attempts at healing, but orthodox medicine brought no help. We began the treatment of Milou in this way:

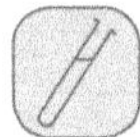

Treatment

20 drops of MMS + 20 drops of acid + 50 mL (0.169 fl oz) water
This tincture was sprayed generously onto the skin 3 times daily for eight weeks. For the following eight weeks we reduced this to 2 times daily. The hair was starting to grow; the improvement was noticeable. We now sprayed two or three times a day for three weeks. At this point in time the winter growth was already so thick that the MMS could no longer penetrate. It already looked very good: Milou was healed, the treatment fully successful. This can be seen in the accompanying pictures. Up to now, nine months on, no new warts have appeared.

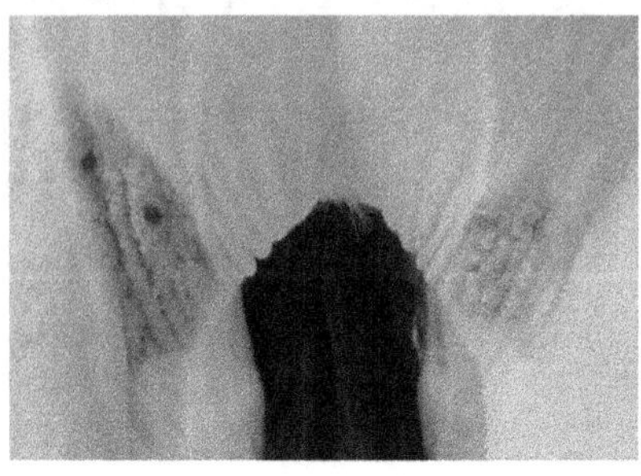
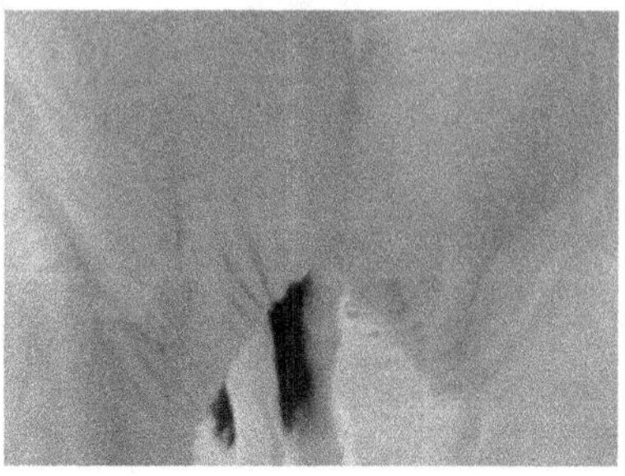

7.3.18 Wound Following a Fall

Description practical example,
report by Ursula W.:

"A horse fell in the morning in the course of long lining and could hardly walk in the evening. The left knee was badly swollen, there was a large abrasion below. The owner brought in a veterinarian from a renowned clinic. The mare received a shot of Epui (pain-relieving, inflammation inhibiting) - that was the treatment in total. All the same, we could see how the whole knee was filling with fluid.

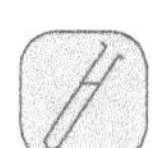

Treatment

I offered to help, and first cleaned the abrasion with hydrogen peroxide. After that I diluted15 drops of MMS activated with dextrogyral lactic acid in 100 mL (3.381 fl oz) sterilized water and applied this to the knee copiously. Then I sprayed on 50% DMSO. After only a few minutes the horse was breathing calmly, allowing itself to be led around the yard without problems. Next day the owner rang to say that the horse was doing splendidly. The wound was dry and the knee was not at all swollen."

7.3.19 Tooth inflammation

See: 7.3.5 EORTH - painful tooth disease

7.4 Rabbit ailments that have been successfully treated with MMS

7.4.1 Abscess

Description practical example:

"Bunny Wolle" came to me with a recurring abscess. A growth in the jaw was repeatedly cut open by the veterinarian and then treated with antibiotics, but the abscess returned again and again.

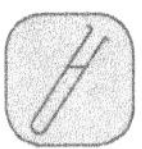

Treatment

1 drop of activated MMS was added to 10mL (0.338 fl oz) water. The rabbit was given 1mL (0.033 fl oz) of this two times daily as well as globules. The intervals between the regrowth became longer until the abscess finally disappeared.

7.4.2 Cheek swollen

Description practical example, report by Conny H.:

"The following is an account of how MMS helped our hare. We drove Hasi with a swollen cheek to the veterinarian who determined that something was biting into its lower jaw. The veterinarian removed a 1 cm (0.393 in) long sliver of wood and informed us that the hare had Actinomycosis."

(Actinomycosis, also called 'lumpy jaw,' is caused by various bacteria.)

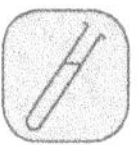

Treatment

"We had to rinse the wound continually as the vet, in order to avoid the lining of the mouth being eaten away, was not able to spray any caustic substances. In the beginning we rinsed with 1 drop of activated MMS in water 3 times a day and sprayed on iodine ointment. Following about five weeks we were down to rinsing 1 time every 1 - 2 days and we then left it to simply grow over. To rinse we employed a syringe to spray the solution on to the wound. Four hands are perhaps an advantage.

I put MMS in the hare's drinking water to this day. In this way we employ no antibiotics, only patience. Actinomycosis is indeed incurable, but Hasi is eating again, and the wound, i.e., the hole, has essentially grown over - there is no festering sore visible.

The veterinarian was most impressed with the effects of MMS of which she had been previously unaware."

7.4.3 Cuniculi

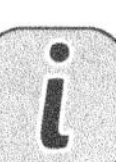

Cuniculi

Encephalitozoon cuniculi (also known as Nosema cuniculi) is a parasitic unicellular, intracellular organism (bacteria) that occurs in the kidneys, brain and other organs. It belongs to phylum Mikrosporidia, the precise systematical function of this parasite is not yet conclusively elucidated ...
(source: Wikipedia, last accessed January 27, 2015)

Description practical example:
"Our female hare could no longer stand, fell over constantly, and had problems with orienting visually. The veterinarian diagnosed European rabbit flea (Encephalitozoon cuniculi),

said that a hare of more than 6½ years should be put to sleep immediately.

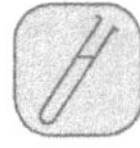

Treatment

I drove home and began the treatment with MMS right away. Mornings and evenings I gave it 4 drops of CDS with a little water directly in the mouth as well as 2 drops of activated MMS mixed in 500 mL (16.907 fl oz) water in her water receptacle. It is now seven-years-old and is fit and healthy. The only remaining indicator of its sickness is a slight lopsidedness of the head. It can live with that without any difficulty."

7.4.4 Cancer

See: "Tumor" 7.4.6

7.4.5 Head Cold

Description practical example:
"My little hare sneezed a lot, and the eyes were full of tears.

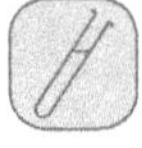

Treatment

"I gave the hare 1 drop of MMS in his water bowl. After three days he seldom sneezed and the eyes were clear. I continued to give him MMS for another week and everything was good. He apparently liked it as his bowl was quickly drunk dry."

7.4.6 Tumor/Cancer

Description practical example 1:
"I did not myself think that MMS would be effective with this illness, and so quickly too! I treated an ulcer (cancer, tumor) affecting my rabbit with CDS, and after only seven days pus/ crust formed and the tumor receded. The tumor was so large

that the mouth was askew. The rabbit was only able to eat finely cut stripes of carrot and was fed by hand. Unaided, he drank only water, if anything. He could now almost chew again, while the tumor was no longer so disturbing![1]

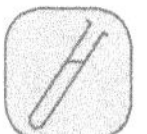

Treatment

The rabbit was given 6 - 8 drops of CDS in its water bowl for 7 days, plus I had it drink directly 2 - 6 drops (likewise increased by the drop) of CDS from a small liquor glass and a small 3 mL (0.101 fl oz) syringe once or twice a day. I found a trick by which it would drink from the syringe: I scratched the animal on the side whereby it would lick involuntarily. In this way it was possible to carefully dispense the full contents of the liquor glass, divided into a number of portions, directly into its mouth. With a little dexterity, it worked well.

The rabbit is very healthy up to now, nothing has reappeared, no more symptoms!"

Description practical example 2:

A hare with a tumor on its stomach was a patient in my practice. For comparison, the tumor was as big as the head (the first picture is Easter 2013 and the second, where the tumor is already much smaller, early June 2013).

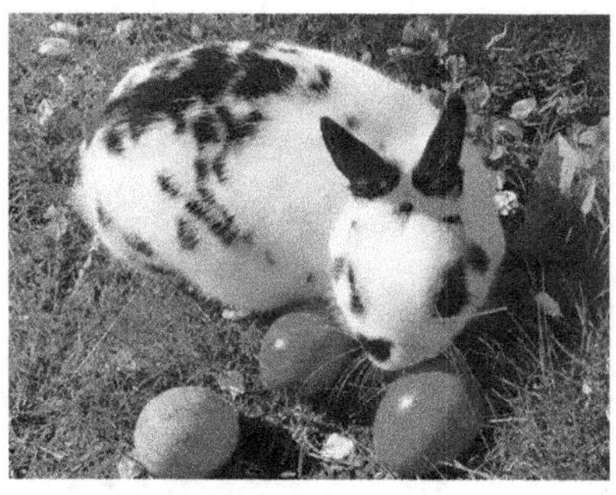
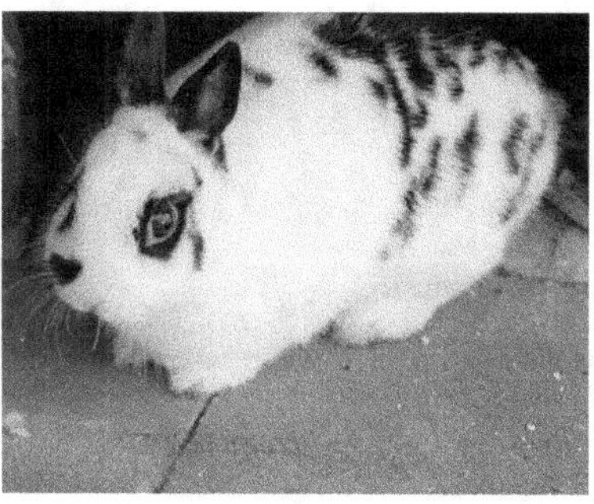

---

1 You can see the whole report along with photos here:
http://www.jim-humble-mms.de/erfolgsfaelle/lebensbedrohlicher-abszess-beim-kaninchen.php

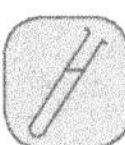

Treatment

The hare was given 2 drops of activated MMS 2 in a little water twice daily direct in the mouth. The tumor retreated further. Since then the hare is doing fine.

7.4.7 Wound on the anus

Description practical example:

A customer came to my practice with her hare. She had seen her miniature hare repeatedly sitting in his drinking bowl. When she looked closely she discovered a small wound on the anus. It looked as though the back passage was inflamed and it smelled disagreeably.

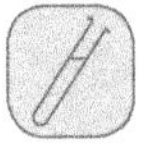

Treatment

The customer gave the hare 2 drops of CDS with some water 3 times daily direct in the mouth.

After only three days there was no more to be seen and the nasty smell was gone. I gave him CDS for another three days. The treatment was most effective, and the hare is now hale and hearty.

7.5 Alpaca maladies that have been successfully treated with MMS

7.5.1 Diarrhea

Description practical example:

Four "new" alpaca joined a customer's herd. Two of the animals suffered from diarrhea. They absolutely refused the medication proffered by the veterinarian.

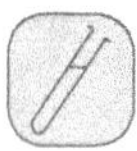

Treatment

So we gave them 20 drops of activated MMS in a 10 L (2.641 gal) bucket to guzzle. Already on the next day the diarrhea had vanished, the excrement looked almost normal. We gave them MMS for another two days; there was no more sign of diarrhea.

7.5.2 Skin Problems

Description practical example:

Following shearing, the owner noticed changes to the skin with scurf and redness on various parts of the body.

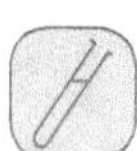

Treatment

We regularly put 20 - 30 drops (approx. 100 mL/3.381 fl oz) of activated MMS in the water trough of approx. 100 L (26.417 gal). After two months there were no more alterations to the skin evident. As a precaution the owner puts 20 drops of MMS in the water every now and then.

7.6 Cow and calf disorders that have been successfully treated with MMS

For cows it is most important to ensure that when preparing Gefeu solution and MMS only hydrochloric acid is used as the activator! The commonplace and at the outset routinely utilized citric acid leads to problems such as diarrhea! Therefore: IMPORTANT! **Use only hydrochloric acid as activator in the case of ruminators!**

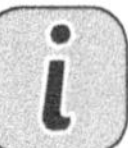

Treatment of cows

As regards treating cows it is essential to note that cows (as well assheep, alpaca) are ruminators. Chlorine dioxide is lost from the activated MMS with each regurgitation. It is imperative that this be accounted for relative to dosage. For me an important factor regarding dosage is the size of the stall. A stall with 30 cows can be dealt with differently than one serving 200 or more. How do I dole MMS out precisely? It would drive any farmer to distraction if I suggested he administer MMS to each cow singly. In isolated cases this is of course possible. Treatment of the whole herd can proceed by means of the water tank. Here too the dosage is crucial. Tests show that CDS dispensed in larger amounts is insufficient when single cows are the frame of reference. We gave individual cows sodium chlorite diluted in water without activator: it is thus first activated by the gastric acid. We obtained impressive results with individual cows employing this method. When we tried this by means of the water tank the outcomes did not satisfy us. The dose that each individual cow receives is apparently not enough.

I am certain that many farmers would confirm that the liver often plays a significant role. Where the problem originates must be regarded. As with pets the feed plays a central role (every farmer knows this of course). To promote healing it is therefore advantageous that cows get to go outside where they can eat fresh grass and herbs. Here too, in relation to large herds, duration is a major factor to consider. With liver problems it can be of benefit to add Swedish bitters or plant tinctures by way of the water tank to strengthen the liver. Dosages must be calculated according to the number of cows.

7.6.1 Abscess

Description practical example,
report from a Swiss farmer:

A cow had an abscess.

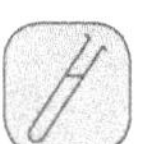

Treatment

10 drops of MMS was dispensed orally with water and without activation 1 time daily, and the region washed with a solution consisting of 20 drops of activated MMS + 500 mL (0.132 fl oz) water. After only a few days it was possible to see how the abscess was shrinking, then opening. The provision of MMS orally continued and the area of the abscess rubbed with Swedish bitters tincture.

Following approximately two weeks it was healed, the cow was well again.

7.6.2 Diarrhea, calves

Description practical example, from a female farmer:

"I often had the problem of calves suffering diarrhea.

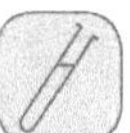

Treatment

I gave them 15 drops of activated MMS once daily with milk out of a bottle.

Since then this issue is history; there is no more diarrhea problem."

7.6.3 Bovine mastitis

Description practical example,
report by C. Thomsen (09.10.2014):

"A cow miscarried on 27.04.2014 on the 117th day of gestation. At this point in time the animal was already in the 198th milking day with an average daily output of about 25 L (6.604 gal). The cow was descended from the bull Lee, a very old bull whose sperm was no longer procurable. It was our explicit aim to maintain this genetic strand in the herd particularly as in the herd of 230 cows only two 'Lee daughters' remained. Subsequent to calving it was paramount that the cow become pregnant again even without semen from bull Lee."

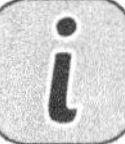

Concerning the use of MMS with dairy herds

"I recommend the utilization of activated MMS with dairy herds especially in relation to expulsion of the afterbirth. If the placenta has not been expelled within 6 - 8 hours of calving we give 20 drops of activated MMS in about 1 L (33.814 fl oz) water to the animal. We divide this in two and express the fluid into the cow's mouth morning and evening with the aid of a bottle. We dispense the appropriate homeopathic medicine as an adjunct. We frequently observe that administering homeopathic medicines in combination with MMS speeds the healing process. The cow is cleared out in a relatively short time."

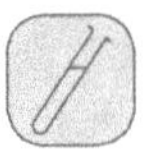

Treatment

We treated the animal in the morning and the evening with 20 drops of MMS as well as the appropriate homeopathic medication. In the middle of May the veterinarian administered Prostaglandin to the cow to thoroughly cleanse (PG: Prostaglandin acts upon the yellow body of the ovary. The animal comes into estrus and cleanses itself as a result). May 31, 2014 we inseminated the animal anew. We decided on a very fecund bull with the express purpose of

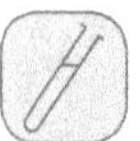

> **Continuation: Treatment**
>
> impregnating the cow. The gravid-analysis on 09.07.2014 was positive. Today (09.10.2014) the cow is in its 131st day of gestation with a milk yield of almost 15 L (3.962 gal)."

7.6.4 Bovine mastitis, milk yield

MMS finds wide application in our operation, including the treatment of bovine mastitis in dairy cattle.

Description practical example 1,
report from C. Thomsen (09.10.2014):

"04.08.2014: In the course of the monthly milk controls milk quantity, cell concentration, fat and protein values for each animal are recorded.

Milk control data of our cow Porsche:

Daily milk yield:	25.6 l (67.765 gal)
Fat content:	3.47
Protein content:	3.03
Cell count:	619

04.08.2014, evening milking:
"Our cow Porsche was afflicted with an acute case of bovine mastitis from one milking to the next. The inflammation broke out directly after the monthly milk controls. The milk yield dropped to less than a Liter (0.264 gal). Her milk had significantly altered in one quarter. The secretion was watery as though running dry. The cow had to be milked into a can. The animal had a cold back; cold, hanging ears; as well as sunken eyes."

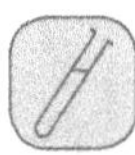

Treatment

"Twice daily we gave her 5 mL (0.169 fl oz/100 drops) of pure sodium chlorite in 0.5 L (16.907 fl oz) water orally, supplemented with homeopathic medicine commensurate with the medication profile. In addition we dispensed 20 mL (0.676 fl oz) CDS in 0.25 L (8.453 fl oz) water 2 times each day, orally.

One week later: Following about a week of this individual treatment the milk yield began to climb slowly. At the end of this week the flow of milk from the sick quarter gradually resumed (a quarter of the udder belongs to each teat), limited though to 1 - 2 L (33.814 - 67.628 fl oz). To the eye it looked like milk again, but now mixed with yellowish flakes. We treated the cow two times a day for two weeks according to this model.

01.09.2014: We performed the milk controls again. Our cow was milked in the pipeline again for the first time.

The milk controls indicate the following values for our cow Porsche.

The initial values are provided in brackets for comparison:

Daily milk yield:	25.8 L (6.815 gal)
Fat content:	4.17 (3.47)
Protein content:	3.16 (3.03)
Cell count:	455 (619)

(Sale of milk with a high cell count is prohibited; such milk must be disposed of!)

Four weeks after the first occurrence of the bovine mastitis the animal's original milk yield was attained. The cell count was down. What caught the eye was that following the treatment the fat-protein quotient was superior. Since then the cow's results are inconspicuous. She runs with the herd and does not require further special treatment."

Here is a table showing the milk controls for comparison:

Date	Daily milk yield	Fat content	Protein content	Cell count
04. 08. 2014	25.6 L (6.762 gal)	3,47	3,03	619
01. 09. 2014	25.8 L (6.815 gal)	4,17	3,16	455
06. 04. 2014	28.05 L (7.410 gal)	4,37	3,33	288

"These figures surprised us. We wish to emphasize that in regard to the homeopathic treatment we very much focused on detoxification of the liver."

Description practical example 2, report from C. Thomsen (09.10.2014):

"The milk yield of our second 'Lee daughter' collapsed from one day to the next. The cell count was very high yet the animal, going by the symptoms, showed no signs of bovine mastitis. This was a very lean, productive cow. The eyes were clear and open, the fur lustrous. The animal had been inseminated to this time. We agreed to treat the animal with MMS. Should the gestation analysis be negative, we would have been obliged to part with the animal. Up to the point when this decision would be made we treated the 'Lee daughter' in accord with Porsche's protocol. The cow repeat bred at one point. I took her to the bulls. The milk yield had stabilized to a degree, at a low level though. Today is the cow's 114th day of gestation with a daily milk yield of 8 L (2.113 gal) on the 479th milking day. Due to the milk yield we will need to administer dry cow therapy early."

Treatment

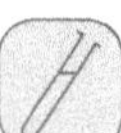

"The cow was very shy and did not like to be touched on the head, still less the dispensation of MMS orally. For this reason we administered MMS directly into the muscle with a dose of 2 mL (0.067 fl oz) CDS 2 times a day in combination with homeopathic substances consistent with the medication profile. After around two weeks the healing process began with the cow."

"Another method of treatment we tried was to inject MMS directly into the affected udder quarter. Right away we had the impression her condition was improved. The consistency of the milk changed positively, the cell count sank. We noted though that long term the milk yield in this quarter was indeed declining gradually. The affected quarter was withering over time. On this basis we applied MMS specifically to treat the quarter that was wasting away. We found a way for the quarter to atrophy stress-free and to give the animal a chance of remaining with the herd.

All things considered, we can determine that the dispensation of MMS orally combined with homeopathic medicines consistent with the pharmaceutical profile is a good option for the treatment of udder ailments. Indeed, we have come to the following conclusion: An intensive and continual program employing MMS is requisite, especially in instances of bovine mastitis. If the treatment is discontinued before the healing process has run its course the animal will regress to its former sickly condition. To repeat a treatment is considerably more time consuming and not as sustainable. When commencing a treatment we ourselves reckon on a duration of approximately four weeks."

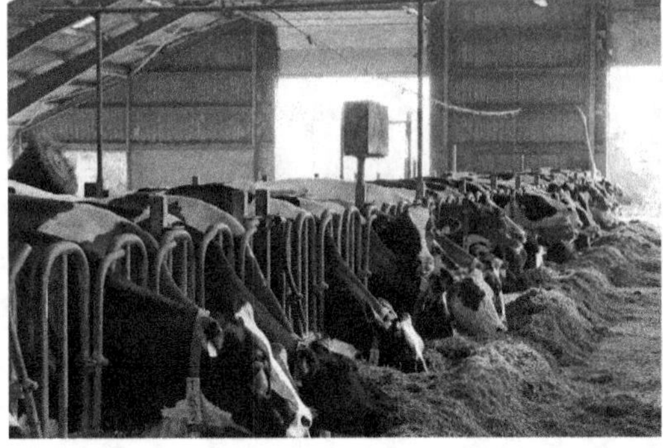 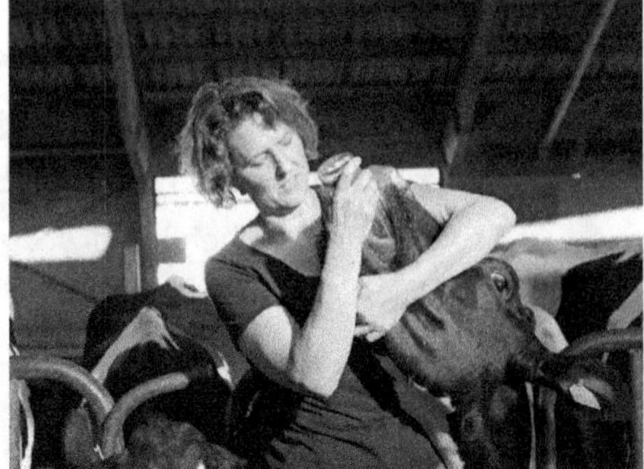

7.7 Assorted animal species, ailments that have been successfully treated with MMS

7.7.1 Mouse with a tumor

Description practical example:
A client noticed one day that blood was running from the eye of the little mouse. By extensive testing with the fingertips I was able to detect a tumor in the region of a muscle in the back of the neck (splenius colli). In addition, the mouse ate little.

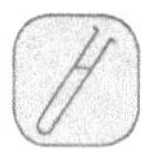

Treatment

The mouse was given 4 drops of CDS in its drinking water over four weeks with the result that the eye cleared, no more blood was to be seen, and the tumor disappeared. Going by his appetite the little mouse is now very well.

7.7.2 Encephalitis, guinea pigs
Encephalitis is an inflammation of the brain.

Description practical example, report by Sylke G:
Guinea pigs with encephalitis can be effectively treated. One should however be careful with the dosage.

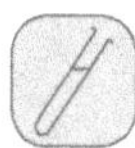

Treatment

I begin with 1 - 2 drops of Gefeu in the drinking water, increasing slowly to 3 - 4 drops. I have noticed in the course of a number of treatments that fully grown animals tolerate larger doses.

7.7.3 Rats

It is necessary to be very careful as regards the dosage with rats. It is advisable to start low rather than to administer too much. The response clearly differs according to age. Older animals often tolerate more drops than younger ones. This certainly relates to their producing vitamin C naturally, and that this production diminishes with age. Here too, extra caution is required.

In the case of fungal infestation there have been good outcomes. By dabbing or painting MMS on externally paralysis of the hindquarters could not only be halted but even improved.

7.7.4 Treatment of Poultry

Fowl have been administered MMS in relation to various problems. A client gave her chick suffering from a cold MMS highly diluted in water and the next day it was already in recovery. Another customer gave MMS to an old chicken that no longer wanted to eat. A day later she was full of life and had again begun to pick.

I have had the same experience with owners of ducks (Indian Runner ducks) who enriched the birds' water with CDS. Improvement could be observed the next day.

I unfortunately possess no diagnoses from veterinarians or specified disorders. I certainly appreciate the engagement of the owners who investigate by putting very small doses (starting with 1 drop of MMS and increasing very gradually) in the drinking water.

Marek's Disease

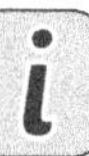

Marek's Disease

(Also known as "visceral leukosis" or "fowl/range paralysis")
Marek's disease is caused by a herpes virus (Gallid Herpesvirus 2).

The virus is produced in the somatic cells or the feather follicles only.
This virus is, among others, related to the human Epstein-Barr virus; domestic fowl are affected mostly.

Description practical example:

A call from a worried woman reached me at the practice. Her rooster had Marek's disease. He tottered, lay about, could not properly attend to his hens; his condition overall was very bad.

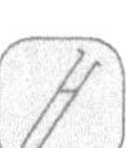

Treatment

We began with 1 drop of CDS 5 times daily. This prescription brought little success at first. The rooster exhibited much the same behavior as before; this was though for me an indication that the medicine was functioning internally.

After about one week the dosage was increased little by little, reaching 4 drops 3 times daily. Recovery came very slowly, but the patience and assurance of the owner paid off and after a few weeks the rooster was proudly running about the garden. As a precaution the hens, ducks and geese that lived with the rooster were administered CDS in the drinking water in ever decreasing amounts. No more problems have arisen since then.

7.7.5 Parakeet with poisoning

Description practical example:
The patient was a parakeet exhibiting symptoms of poisoning.

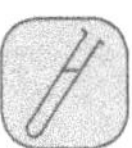

Treatment

With the aid of a pipette I fed the little parakeet 1 drop of CDS mixed in a tiny amount of water a number of times a day. That evening he was already sitting perkily on his perch.

8 Complementary Remedies

*O*ne could assuredly catalog myriads of remarkable help-ers with respect to the healing of humans and animals. The palette is large and is growing continually. Very old knowledge corroborates most medications. Often these are, as already revealed, prohibited by means of subtle rationales and interdictions.

There are many remarkable helpers in relation to the healing of humans and animals.

And certainly yet more amazing substances are in existence. You will find further information about these in the Internet. I wish you an abundance of joy in the discovering!

To follow I describe a number of complementary substances I employ in in my animal-care practice.

8.1 DMSO

DMSO (chemical formula C_2H_6OS) is something of a "misjudged universal remedy." DMSO celebrated its 140th birthday in 2006. The substance was first synthesized in 1866 by the Russian scientist Alexander Saytzeff who published his discovery in a German science journal in 1867.

DMSO: a "misconstrued wonder drug"

It was not until 1961, almost one hundred years later, that its medicinal potentials were recognized. Dr. Stanley Jacob of the Oregon Health Sciences University was actually seeking a suitable substance for the conservation of organs designated for transplantation as he one day discovered that this clear, musty liquid, smelling faintly of garlic was readily able to penetrate and be thoroughly absorbed by human skin. Jacob began to experiment and soon found that he was evidently dealing with a multifaceted active agent.

Dr. Stanley Jacob discovered the therapeutic uses of DMSO in 1961.

Due to its reputation as a "miracle cure" the Food and Drug Administration (FDA) tested DMSO. The FDA determined

Food and Drug Administration (FDA)

that it had the adverse effect of causing shortsightedness in swine, dogs and rabbits when applied in high doses (the amount is not known). This assertion brought about an interim standstill for DMSO in 1965.

Shortsightedness as concerns humans has never been substantiated. And thus far I have not heard of an incidence in the case of animals; hence I cannot verify this!

A germane extract from the book "DMSO: Nature's Healer" by Dr. Morton Walker:

DMSO: Employed as a strong pain killer

The American Medical Association (AMA) held a leadership conference the weekend of February 14, 1981, and one of the speakers was Otis R. Bowen, M.D. Dr. Bowen is former governor of Indiana, a leader in medicine, management, and politics. In his presentation to the AMA he shocked the assembly by admitting that he took the law into his own hands and used an illegal drug to ease his wife's pain while she was dying. Beth Bowen died January 1, 1981 following months of agony from multiple myeloma, a type of bone cancer.

Dr. Bowen, who was preparing to step down from the governorship at the time, turned to Dimethyl sulfoxide, i.e., DMSO, to ease his wife's intense pain. He had obtained the liquid solvent from a veterinarian and found that it relieved his wife's suffering "in minutes." The Food and Drug administration (FDA) forbids the use of DMSO in humans except when treating a rare urinary bladder condition. Even in the face of the government ban Dr. Brown did what he knew was right for his wife by administering DMSO intravenously. "Why can't dying persons with severe pain have easy prescription access?" he asked in his speech. "The only explanation I could find was that, in dogs only, after prolonged use and heavy dosage it caused an occasional cataract." Here I would like to point out that in practice DMSO has already been intravenously administered many times. In none of these treatments did a cataract develop. Quite the oppo-site: In the case of older dogs an improvement in visual acuity was observed! Here too, the quantity makes the poison.

Before you've read very far into this book, you'll probably be asking questions similar to Dr. Bowen's. It won't be difficult to identify with the patients involved, some of whom have been forced to take treat-ment into their own hands by turning to DMSO. DMSO has, in fact, not been found to be unsafe for humans; any side effects are minor irritations."

The virtues of DMSO

"DMSO stops bacterial growth. It relieves pain. As a vasodilator, the drug enlarges small blood vessels, increasing the circulation to a region. It softens scar tissue and soothes burns.

DMSO's anti-inflammatory activity relieves the swelling and inflammation of arthritis, bursitis, tendinitis, and other musculoskeletal injuries. And it does many more good things of a therapeutic nature for anyone who is injured or ill."

Nina Hawranke published an excellent article in Nexus 24 / August - September 2008. Here is a short extract:

"... That the pharmaceutical industry shows no great interest in this substance is easy to explain. On the one hand, the broad palette of ailments against which DMSO is effective is undoubtedly of conse-quence, it competes with many in-house products. On the other, DMSO is not only utilized pharmacologically but also industrially

and cannot be patented - that is not an attractive attribute as regards marketing strategy. Many concerns defend themselves by claiming that there are plenty of products that yield the same outcomes. Terry Bristol, PhD, President of the Institute for Science, Engineering and Public Policy in Portland, Oregon, who supported Stanley Jacob during his researches, views the advantages though as being with DMSO:

"DMSO is much less toxic than other substances, and has fewer side effects."

According to the therapeutic index DMSO is indeed seven times safer than aspirin. The only side effects observed thus far are a garlicky odor and irritation of the skin with some individuals, which Walker attributes to dehydration of the skin, and which after a number of applications disappears. Regardless, DMSO fumes ought not be inhaled. DMSO injected intravenously can occasionally lead to headaches. Toxicity or carcinogenic effects could not be experimentally verified."

In the pivotal book (See: Margin notes) about DMSO by Dr. Hartmut Fischer, published by Daniel-Peter-Verlag, you will find the following information (p. 237 - 238):

"DMSO is a natural product derived from wood.

The across the board healing power of DMSO is without equal, and ought to be regarded as a preeminent fundament of therapy. DMSO is not interchangeable, possessing a staggeringly wide palette of congruous qualities.

... For animals, it is primarily applied externally to treat disorders of the musculoskeletal system, especially the limbs. Inflamed joints, injuries, swelling, strains, and many other ailments affecting domestic, sports, and service animals can be treated most effectively on one's own initiative with DMSO. For the limbs a 60 - 70% dilution can be prepared. Drops (sterile solutions!) can likewise be administered externally for disorders of the ears, nose and eyes.

Further possible applications for highly concentrated, aqueous DMSO solution are the washing of wounds, festering sores, abscesses, and fistulas. The 50 - 80% mixture can be administered directly into the affected opening with the aid of a plastic dropper bottle or plastic syringe.

... Ingestion of DMSO is also practicable when treating muscle, joint, and bone ailments. Indeed, all kinds of animal disorders can be treated in this manner ...

The smell and flavor are odd for an animal, hence creativity is called for when administering orally."

DMSO for inflamed joints, injuries, swelling, sprains ...

These are only a few extracts from the DMSO Handbook. For me, DMSO often acts as a "door opener." It opens up, so to say, the path to the blood and musculature. Medicines such as MMS/CDL or tinctures can thus penetrate the tissue faster and deeper so the healing process is swifter. With open hot spots or wounds I dab the region with a mixture of MMS/CDL and water, and then spray on some 50% DMSO solution.

DMSO assists in conveying medicine to the seat of the condition.

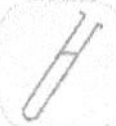

Dosage

A mixture of equal parts CDL and DMSO diluted in water (e.g., 10 mL [3.381 fl oz] CDL/CDLplus + 10 mL [3.381 fl oz] DMSO + 10 mL [3.381 fl oz] water) has proven to be very effective for treating open wounds. Draw this into a syringe and flush out the wound. In this way the bacteria can be combated locally and the healing process accelerated.

DMSO in combination with a comfrey tincture is also effectual when handling joint pain, or for instance when a dog has a dislocation: I rub 50% DMSO solution into the area and then comfrey tincture. When inflammation is suspected I dispense MMS or CDL/CDLplus orally.

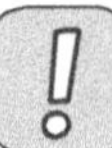

Please don't be dismayed when administering DMSO that the animals begin to smell "off." The odor resembles garlic. I often give my animals DMSO along with CDL/CDLplus and cottage cheese or natural yoghurt to mask the smell. The cats are delighted each time they get a special treat.

A positive secondary effect of DMSO taken orally is that ticks are repelled: It seems these plaguing spirits do not appreciate the smell of garlic. Where possible, DMSO applied externally in a greater than 50% solution should first be spot-tested as reactions such as itching or reddening may occur; I have never detected such when applying a 50% solution.

8.2 Swedish Bitters

Here is an extract from Wikipedia (January 28, 2015) regarding the history of Swedish Bitters:

"The name derives from the nationality of the Swedish medics and chemists Klaus Samst and Urban Hjärne. Urban Hjärne had a laboratory on Kungsholmen where he prepared 'secret' potions. In 1692 he received permission to sell Amarum through apothecaries. The doctor Klaus Samst is thought to have rediscovered the formula in the 18th Century. It had earlier been known by the Samst family, and then forgotten. The Swiss-German Theophrastus Bombastus von Hohenheim, designated Paracelsus, is to have developed a similar medicine in the 16th Century. The Austrian herbalist Maria Treben popularized Swedish bitters with her 1980 bestseller 'Gesundheit aus der Apotheke Gottes' (Health Through God's Pharmacy)."

Swedish Bitters: An important medicine for support of the metabolism and fortification of the immune system

The famous herbalist Maria Treben knew the merits of Swedish bitters; she viewed it to truly be a miracle elixir. I must say though, I battle with the bitter taste of this mixture; even diluted in water it shakes me time and again. Regardless of how my stomach rebels, still I imbibe it enthusiastically - before long the gut is calm.

Maria Treben appreciated the merits of Swedish bitters.

Animals respond quite differently.

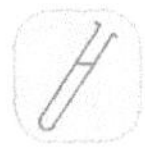

> **Dosage**
>
> Dilute ½ - 1 teaspoon in warm water for dogs according to size. Horses can be given Swedish bitters pure (1 tablespoon) or diluted in water and poured onto the food. Horses love this bitter concoction - it is amusing to see how eager they get.

It is an important means of support for the metabolism. Swedish bitters fortify the immune system and more. Swedish bitters alleviates gastrointestinal tract disorders. It is fascinating how wide-ranging the application of Swedish bitters is, and the profusion of symptoms it soothes.

Say a dog has a skin problem: I treat this externally with MMS, and the root, the metabolism, with Swedish bitters. Of course this differs from animal to animal and must always be tested out.

8.3 Zeolite

Zeolites possess outstanding detoxifying qualities and are an ideal complement to MMS.

Zeolites are crystalline aluminosilicates that appear in nature in numerous modifications. Zeolites are derived from fine-ground lava and have detoxifying capacities akin to sponges. They are an ideal supplement to MMS. MMS deactivates viruses, bacteria, and pathogens in the organism; zeolites, like a dump truck, remove the hazardous waste. They absorb poisons in the body, while providing key minerals. It is clear to see that in combination with zeolite the effect of MMS is increased many times over.

Our organism is more and more frequently confronted with poisonous metals such as mercury, palladium, cadmium, lead, nickel, et cetera. Apart from the immune system these materials stress the liver, kidneys, and intestines. These can enter the body through food, medicines, vaccinations, and water. Often our animals take them in without our noticing.[1]

Animals ingest poisons unnoticed.

It is a terrific help expunging bacteria, viruses, fungi and parasites devitalized by MMS/CDL/CDLplus. So, during the day I dispense MMS/CDL/CDLplus in small doses and zeolite to channel in the evening. The process of recovery is promoted without the metabolism and liver being excessively stressed: The liver performs its functions at night.

Zeolite is an efficient channel for poisons.

Attributes that make zeolite clinoptilolites so worthwhile in comparison to other minerals:
- the enormous active surface area resulting in tremendous absorbance of poisons, especially extra-fine pulverized zeolite (2 micrometer or 2000 nanometer);
- the unique mineral honeycomb structure; and
- the abundance of applications.

Zeolite underpins and assists in the bodily processes of detoxification and elimination in that it binds toxic elements by means of selective ion exchange and adsorption (enhancement) as well as filtering larger unphysiological particles through the molecular sieve. The organism is thus provided with essential biogenic minerals like calcium (Ca), magnesium (Mg), sodium (Na), potassium (K) and silicon dioxide (SiO2).

Zeolite provides the organism with essential minerals such as calcium, magnesium, sodium, potassium and silicon dioxide.

---

1   Read more: http://www.zentrum-der-gesundheit.de/ schwer-metalle-ausleiten-ia.htmL#ixzz313dBRRfi (27. 01. 2015).

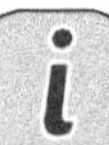

> ## Attributes of zeolite
>
> **A range of publications credit the following attributes to Zeolite:**
>
> - Zeolite channels environmental poisons, storage poisons, and heavy metals from the intestines and sluices them from the body.
> - Zeolite absorbs poisons that accumulate in the body due to bacteria, fungi, over-acidity, fermentation, and putrescence.
> - Zeolite supports intestinal activity and the immune system.
> - Zeolite reduces stress and protects cells from free radicals.
> - Zeolite obviates premature aging.
> - Zeolite disburdens the liver, the kidneys, the connective tissue, and the skin.
> - Zeolite improves the nourishment of the body and the resorption of essential nutrients and minerals.
> - Zeolite improves the supply to the body of antioxidants and functions like an antirust agent.
> - Zeolite is the single known agent that binds radioactive emissions to itself and can actually rid the body of such (Cookies containing zeolite were fed to children in Chernobyl with great success.) Zeolite does not metabolize, therefore overdosage is practically impossible. Zeolite, along with contaminates and toxins, is totally eliminated in 24 hours.

The greater the clinoptilolite content in zeolite, the better the quality.

Drinking sufficient water reinforces the cleansing powers of activated zeolite. The positive effects are so diverse that currently a comprehensive study of clinoptilolite zeolite as a basis therapeutic agent for the treatment of numerous chronic conditions, including allergies, fungus and tumor diseases, is in progress.

It is important to note: According to Dr. Hartmut Fischer no oxidants should be taken (MMS/CDL) without supplying the body with zeolite (with a 4 hour time offset). Zeolite is a powerful antioxidant, absorbing poisons. It is advisable to dispense MMS in the morning and afternoon and zeolite in the evening.

> ## Dosage of zeolite for animals
>
> The dose can be divided in two. The following is a rule of thumb, not a precept! Mostly I do it this way: Cats and small dogs - 1 knifepoint; big dogs - 1 teaspoon; horses - 1 tablespoon. It is essential to first stir the powder in with a little water, and then mix the brew in with the meal.
>
> | | Morning | Evening |
> |--------|---------------|---------------|
> | **Cat** | 1 knifepoint | 1 knifepoint |
> | **Dog** | 1 teaspoon | 1 teaspoon |
> | **Horse** | 1 tablespoon | 1 tablespoon |

8.4 Bentonite

Bentonite is a healing earth with exceptional powers. Its chief merits are the absorption of toxins from the alimentary system and the harmonizing of the gastrointestinal milieu, in turn promoting the development of healthy intestinal flora and thereby activating the self-healing forces of the organism.[1]

Bentonite - A healing earth with exceptional powers

The mineral-rich clay bentonite is a completely natural substance with many positive attributes. I would like to highlight two of these today: Its effect on diarrhea, and its wide-ranging detoxifying qualities that help protect the whole body from toxins and noxious substances of all kinds.

Bentonite is a completely natural substance.

---

1   More under: http://www.zentrum-der-gesundheit.de/ bentonit-wahrheit-ia.htmL#ixzz313eja9FG (17.01.2015).

Great adsorptive capability.

Bentonite is a clay formed by the weathering of volcanic ash. Bentonite is pulverized very fine, and its surface area is thus very large. Its ions are negatively charged. These characteristics lend it unusually high adsorptive capabilities.

8.4.1 Detoxification with the mineral clay bentonite

Bentonite reduces harmful substances in the body limiting the burden on the emunctory organs: Liver, kidneys, and intestines.

Adsorption through mineral clays is an efficient means of detoxification. Adsorption is the process by which bentonite attracts and holds materials and particles to its surface. When this occurs in the human digestive system these substances are not reabsorbed. Thus they do not enter the bloodstream, but are due to bentonite eliminated with the stool. Detox or intestinal cleansing programs are therefore more effective when the mineral clay bentonite is involved.

Bentonite can also be employed as a course of treatment, but functions exceptionally well as a natural healing medicine taken in small amounts each day to bind and dispose of the contaminants that derive from the environment and nutrients. The burden on the body due to contaminants is thereby limited; the emunctories (liver, kidneys, intestines) are on the one hand relieved while the health is protected and improved overall. Which contaminates are adsorbed and then discarded?

Bentonite binds harmful bacteria, heavy metals, residual pesticides, mildew poisons, and radioactive particles. Bentonite acts in the intestines in the main, hence its capacity to hold bacteria is especially useful in combating bacterial intestinal disorders.

8.4.2 Bentonite: The ideal diarrhetic medicine

Conventional diarrhetic medications do not offer what one might desire - they potentially lead to further complications by blocking the intestines and thus retaining the bacteria. A substance that does not simply paralyze the intestines, but supports their ability to self-heal instead is to be preferred.

Bentonite augments the capacity of the body to heal itself.

The ideal diarrhetic medication ought achieve the following:

- Reduce the count of bacteria through adsorption and dispose of harmful bacteria;
- Adsorb and channel bacterial toxins;
- Absorb excess liquid;
- Augment stool formation;
- Adsorb gas;
- Restore healthy intestinal flora;
- ... and all of this WITHOUT incapacitating the gastro-intestinal peristalsis or having damaging side effects.

Bentonite fulfills these criteria due to its large surface area and powerful adsorption capabilities. This mineral laden clay is therefore highly recommended as natural first-aid in the event of diarrhea and belongs in every first-aid kit.

Natural first-aid for diarrhea.

At the practice I frequently dispense bentonite to follow treatment with MMS/CDL/CDLplus and zeolite in order to promote the growth and revitalization of animals' intestinal flora.

The dosage of bentonite is the same as zeolite. Here too, stir the powder into a little water and mix this brew in with the food.

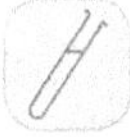

Dosage

This dosage may be dispensed singly, or divided in two. This is a guide and not a prescription! Mostly I do it like this: Cats and small dogs - 1 knifepoint, big dogs - 1 teaspoon, horses 1 - tablespoon.

It is important to stir the powder into a little water and mix the brew in with the food.

	Morning	Evening
Cat	1 knifepoint	1 knifepoint
Dog	1 teaspoon	1 teaspoon
Horse	1 tablespoon	1 tablespoon

8.5 Plant tinctures - phytotherapy

There are multitudes of medicinal herbs in our Latitude. These days many people consider them to be "weeds." Already as a child I came to know these wonderful helpers through my parents. Comfrey tincture and English marigold salve, self-made naturally, were always at the ready.

Self-produced herbal medicines are valuable aids to healing.

Sad that so much of this old knowledge is being forgotten. Fortunately there are engaged people such as my friend Sabine who are "unearthing" this knowledge, about plants for instance, aiding me greatly in my work. For that I am most thankful.

My mother told me that the farmers used to give comfrey to the pigs to prevent swine erysipelas.

For years I have been producing tinctures and salves from medicinal herbs that I have mostly collected myself. I have first dabbed inflamed ears with MMS and then rubbed on a salve of ground ivy and marigold. The outcomes are inspiring. New tinctures, mixtures and salves are continually being added to my assortment.

I choose local plants as these can be obtained fresh where possible. I avoid using plants from virgin forest or the like - the long-distance delivery is not to my liking. The cultivated areas in many lands are heavy with pesticides, especially conspicuous with ginseng: when genuinely clean, unadulterated quality is required it generally very expensive. I find a great deal of the herbs on our pasture or on holiday in the Bavarian Almwiese (Mountain Meadows). Here too: Each of us must oneself decide whether or not to use these with their animals!

Application of local plants preferable

Tinctures help me in marvelous ways when dealing with psychological problems. Angelica, chicory, daisies and many other gifts from Mother Nature aid me in my work with animals. The daisy is a wonderful "antidepressant," restoring joy to living. Angelica brings among other things self-confidence and trust.

Every plant has mental and physical aspects. Angelica, on the bodily plane, can help with gastrointestinal problems. Of course it is best to find a therapist who works with plant-based healing and performs tests to ascertain the suitable plant for your animal.

In my practice I frequently use MMS for the bodily problems and plant tinctures for the psychological, harmonizing the physical and the mental - the process of healing is speedier.

Without doubt you are asking: Where do I come by comfrey tincture, or daisy tincture, or angelica tincture?
Well, my counsel is: Make your own! Of course there is loads to buy, though you will save a great deal of money, and it's fun, going out into nature to look for plants.

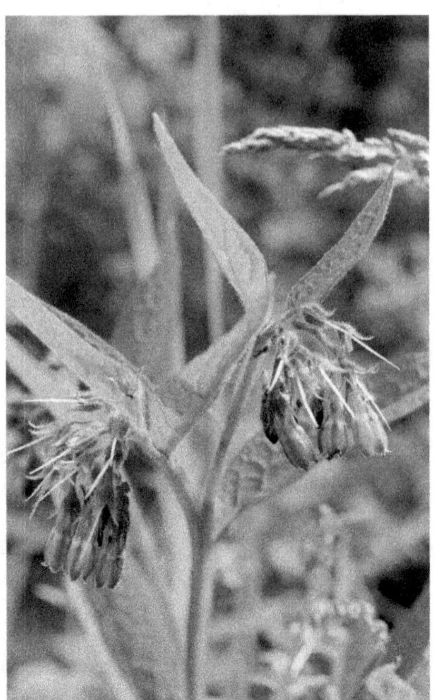

Comfrey

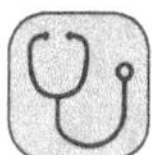

Preparing a daisy tincture

The daisy grows on many lawns and in parks. Pick a few blooms, place them in a screw jar, cover in alcohol (vodka, gin), and place the glass on the windowsill. It should stand there for about four weeks - a lunar cycle (28 days) it's said. Occasionally shake the glass: In alchemic laboratories such formulations are normally turned clockwise every morning at sunrise, and anti-clockwise every evening when the moon comes up.

At the end of 28 days the liquid is poured into a glass or phial; paste a label on ... done!

Some medicinal herbs can be bought dried. To forage oneself, to pluck or to grub out, bestows this process, I find, greater healing powers. I love this work. In our neighborhood they call me "The Bavarian Herb Witch" - truly a great honor!

Dried herbs can also be used.

8.6 OPC - The active ingredient in grape seed extract

OPC was discovered by the French scientist and professor Jack Masquelier subsequent to the Second World War. OPC, and its weaker form Terrakraft, functions like a kind of fountain of youth for the body. OPC is a polyphenol, a large grouping of secondary plant matter.

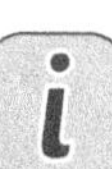

What is OPC?

OPC - the abbreviation for "oligomeric proanthocyanidinis" is an extract of red wine grape seeds. It can be taken daily in capsule form: "one tanks up on sun daily, and the full powers of the vineyard!" says Robert Franz. That grape seeds are so

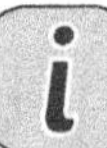

Continuation: What is OPC?

wholesome was discovered some sixty years ago - but to this day this is ignored by Medicine (the pharmaceutical industry), with good reason, as Robert Franz repeatedly highlights: "If everyone took OPC the pharmaceutical industry would suffer huge losses of profit."[1]

Moreover, that a glass of red wine is healthy is widely known - red wine is made from grapes and therefore contains the active agent OPC. With OPC the benefits of many glasses of wine can be enjoyed without developing an alcohol problem. OPC can be given to our animals without concern; alcohol is particularly dangerous for cats. I find OPC to be very helpful when treating weakened, sick animals. Likewise, it can bring the metabolism back in play when needed. Another virtue of OPC is that it gently channels harmful substances. OPC is a natural nutritional supplement.

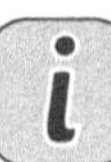

OPC and its healing properties

OPC is a plant-based antioxidant. OPC ought not be used simultaneously with MMS, CDL and CDLplus as the substances cancel one another out. It is advisable to cleanse with MMS/CDL and then build up the body with OPC to follow - a gap of at least four hours between the dispensing of MMS/CDL and OPC should be observed. Grape seed extract has an extraordinarily positive effect on the following organs and illnesses:

Heart, vessels, blood, diabetes, allergies, skin, connective tissue, injuries, degenerative aging phenomena, respiratory passages, mood, immune system, kidneys. It is a recognized backup for all modes of healing.

---

1 This book by Robert Franz is very good as regards this topic: "The Fundament of Human Health" (Das Fundament menschlicher Gesundheit), Otto-LutzVerlag.

8.7 Borax

The chemical designation of Borax is Sodium borate. Borax is a natural mineral that unfortunately is found rarely. One way it is constituted is by the drying up of salt lakes. It exists in crystalline and solid forms.

Boron: A naturally occurring mineral

Boron is an important component in nature. Unfortunately the reserves of this important mineral have for many years been depleted and therefore foodstuffs contain hardly any or no boron. Our bodies are thus boron deficient. What are the effects of this deficiency in the body?

The boron component in foodstuffs has reduced significantly.

Implications of Boron Deficiency

Boron deficiency gives rise to hyperactivity of the parathyroid gland, an excess of hormones is released. These hormones in turn drain calcium from the bones and teeth. The calcium level increases in the blood potentially leading to osteoarthritis (arthrosis) of the joints, osteoporosis, and dental problems. With oncoming age high calcium levels cause calcification of the soft tissue giving rise to muscle tension and stiffening joints. Arteries and the endocrine glands, especially the pineal gland, calcify. Final outcome: Kidney stones, calcification of the kidneys, kidney failure. These problems are common with our animals.

Another important point: Due to diet and inoculation et cetera, we supply a great deal of aluminum to the body. Like in a contest, one aluminum molecule

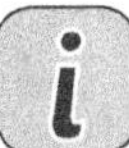

Continuation: Implications of Boron Deficiency

displaces three boron molecules. In that we provide more aluminum than boron to the bodies of our animals we can discount there being any "contest."

Borax offers more positive consequences in relation to disorders such as osteoarthritis, cancer, and more: Arthritis and joint complaints are not to be overlooked.

Administering borax together with magnesium is most effective. Take care administering borax! Too much can be harmful!

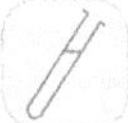

Borax dosage

(This is the dosage for humans averaging 70 kg (154.324 lb). This must be converted to suit our animals.)

Normal dose: We dissolve 1 lightly heaped teaspoon (5 - 6 g / 0.176 - 0.211 oz) in 1 L (33.814 fl oz) fresh water in a bottle.

Take 1 - 2 teaspoons of this concentrate daily.

A dog of approximately 35 kg (77.161 lb) would be given ½ - 1 teaspoon daily. A teaspoon equals 5 mL (0.169 fl oz).

Assuming that a person of approximately 70 kg (154.323 lb) receives 10 mL (2 teaspoons/0.338 fl oz), then a dog weighing 20 kg (44.092 lb) would be given 2.8 mL (0.094 fl oz).

Borax, as are so many things, is prohibited in Germany and is thus difficult to obtain. Borax can be ordered in England via the Internet. If you decide for this option be sure that you order pure borax. Here in Germany, to prevent oral intake, borax is often mixed with harmful substances.

It is astounding to read of all these "alternative" medicines and then to arrive at the same conclusion: They are inexpensive, helpful, and on stitched-together grounds are forbidden or simply disappeared by the WHO and similar institutions where vast sums of money are generated by way of pharmaceuticals.

8.8 Mumijo

Mumijo, called Shilajit in some regions, is a natural product that has been used for healing and fortification for thousands of years in Central Asian folk medicine, and has a permanent place in Ayurvedic medicine. Mumijo is deployed to handle many disorders, the metabolic processes along with others.

Mumijo is a standby in Ayurvedic medecine.

Despite thorough botanical and geological analysis of the respective deposits there is no definitive explanation as to the exact process of formation that can also vary according to location. What is endorsed by science is that the prerequisite conditions that apply to all deposits are: A long period of intensive insolation (solar radiation), that the air is exceptionally clean, and specific vegetation. Above all succulents, especially of the Euphorbia genus, are required for the formation of the atypically water-soluble mumijo latex. (Source: Wikipedia, 25.01.2015)

Long and intensive insolation (solar radiation) - an important precondition for the genesis of Mumijo

In the book "Mumijo, Black Gold of the Himalayas" by Dr. Wolfgang Widmann the following dosages are recommended for humans weighing approximately 70 kg (154.324 lb):

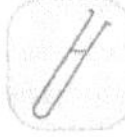

Mumijo - Dosage

1. Between 50 and 800 mg (0.00176 - 0.028 oz) of mumijo can be taken daily without harm.
2. A dose of 200 mg (0.007 oz) is optimal.
3. The schedule is variable according to the disorder. A standard dose of 2 - 3 times daily is recommended.
4. Mumijo is bile expelling with dosages of 200 mg (0.007 oz).

These indications are for humans weighing approximately 70 kg (154.323 lb). Dosage for specific animals must be recalculated according to weight. Once again: Less is often more!

8.9 Moringa oleifera

Moringa oleifera is known as the "Miracle Tree."

Moringa is called "The Miracle Tree." Moringa contains 18 of 20 amino acids that are important in relation to the transport of oxygen, brain function, and concentration. Over 700 studies confirm the multi-dimensional promotion of health by the tree, leaves, and fruit. The leaves especially have an astounding antioxidizing effect.

Studies credit antioxidizing and manifold healing properties to the tree, leaves, and fruit.

Moringa Oleifera powder should be added to the feed of animals with immunodeficiencies, skin problems, bone and joint problems, problems with digestion, metabolic disorders, itch, developmental disorders, halitosis, and unhealthy and lusterless fur.

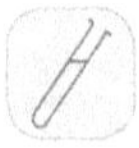

Moringa oleifera dosage

Feeding recommendation: For a dog of 20 kg (44.092 lb) dispense a heaped knifepoint. Animals of other weights receive less or more accordingly.

Barbara Simonsohn and Joachim Funk describe applications for animals in their book "Moringa, The Edible Miracle Tree" (Moringa, der essbare Wunderbaum).

Our pets, as we know, are not invulnerable to illness and being overweight - Moringa is endowed with impressive attributes. For example, the authors tell of administering moringa to overwrought horses that frighten with every rustle and subsequently become more self-confident and composed.
Our animals' immune system is reinforced by moringa, it is an effective back-up in cases of viral illness. Moringa can be dispensed to animals daily with the feed, resulting in luminous eyes and shining fur. Digestion and detoxification are promoted, function properly in the shortest time.

Moringa oleifera fortifies the immune system and even promotes self-confidence and composure with our animals.

As with humans, moringa can help in cases of arthritis, osteoporosis, high blood pressure, cancer, and rheumatism. There are even more disorders where moringa is of assistance: Sight is conserved, and dogs suffering hip dysplasia can be helped. Moringa due to its remarkable aggregation of vital substances can aid in dogs and cats losing weight.

In the USA and Great Britain there are treatment centers for overweight cats and dogs. It is estimated that in the USA alone there are four million overweight dogs; five percent of American dogs are obese. Aside from exercise, food rich in vital substances is the remedy for obesity. Slimming pills for pets (e.g. "Slentrol") are already standard in the USA, but as with humans these have considerable side effects.

Help with our overweight animals

Not only do sick animals and their keepers suffer, but for all those concerned a visit to the veterinarian costs money, strength, and nerves. All that you have read about the health benefits of moringa for humans goes for animals as well: fertility increases, pregnancy is lighter, nursing mothers produce enough quality mother's milk, and the immune system

Moringa oleifera fortifies the immune system, increases fertility, and eases pregnancy.

is bolstered. Animals that receive moringa are simply fitter, more vital, and healthier, which is clear to see as well: Bright eyes, shining fur.

Small animals receive a knifepoint with their food, larger animals accordingly more.

Moringa oleifera also helps deer.

Moringa even helps deer; these animals also become, fitter, more cheerful, and less often sick. Fish suffer no more fungal infestation. (Based on: "Moringa, The Edible Miracle Tree" (Moringa, der essbare Wunderbaum) by Barbara Simonsohn and Joachim Funk)

Exchange of experiences: Moringa oleifera and various animals - these reports are abstracted from the book "Moringa, The Edible Miracle Tree" (Moringa der essbare Wunderbaum)

Alsatian dog

Example 1: Helga Vogel

"I have been working in an animal shelter for 14 years. I have given the animals moringa there as well. An old Alsatian spent his twilight free of ailments. A Rottweiler and a mongrel had shiny fur and astounding levels of fitness.

Likewise, Egon the deer received his moringa. Each time change of coat arrived Egon was enfeebled. With the onset of age he coped less and less. Thanks to moringa these ailments are of the past."

Longhaired tomcat

Example 2: Christian Kaliauer from Aschach on the Danube

"Hello, my name is Benni. I am a five-year-old, white, longhaired tomcat. Four weeks ago my master began mixing some kind of green stuff in my food once a day. At first I thought: 'He's nuts! What, as a cat, should I do with green stuff when I love mice, frogs and birds above all!' Still, after a week I noticed something strange: all at once no mouse could escape me! And my master thought that I had grown lots of beautiful fur, and the tears in my eyes totally dis-

appeared. When I observed what good it did my master to take moringa as well, I decided instantly that I would from now on eagerly devour this green stuff and recommend it to all the cats in my neighborhood."

Example 3: Peter

Peter was looking for a new ingredient for his shrimp feed. "I set up a stick with moringa for my catfish. What can I say: All the animals in the aquarium fly to this stick at feeding time. Not only catfish, but prawns, crabs, snails, and other fish. My partner has a dog. Her dog is fed a knifepoint each morning. The dog is fourteen-years of age and is currently enjoying his second spring!"

Fish

Example 4: Angelika

"Our dog, a West Highland White Terrier, was apathetic, halfhearted, and very sleepy. The fur was mangy and the veterinarian had no suggestions. I mixed moringa powder in with the food. Within fourteen days the dog was transformed. He sprang about, barked joyously again, and his fur was smooth and lustrous."

West Highland White Terrier

Example 5: Hansjörg Stübler

Hansjörg lives on Moorea Maharepa, an island neighboring Tahiti and cares for injured dogs and cats, often struck by cars. My home remedy for open wounds is a mixture of a green healing earth 'Argile verte' (green clay = bentonite) from France and moringa powder. The mixture is made up of three parts healing earth to one part moringa. I have treated wounds where one seriously considered putting the animal down. Simply mix, add a little water to produce a brew, and then rub on carefully. When it is not possible to rub the mixture on I pour it straight onto the wound."

Moringa oleifera on open wounds

8.10 Colloidal silver

Colloidal silver can be employed as an effective natural antibiotic.

Hundreds of years before the pharmaceutical industry developed many illnesses were treated with a single medicine in particular: Colloidal silver. The virtue of colloidal silver is that it is extremely effective in combating bacteria, viruses, and fungi. It is able to kill off, within the shortest time and without side effects, up to 650 different pathogenic agents, and can be employed as a natural antibiotic.

In medieval times for instance silver cutlery was used in order to eliminate bacteria.

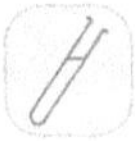

Dosage	
Cats, small dogs , hares and rabbits	5 mL (0.169 fl oz) 5 - 25 ppm solution 2 x daily
Big dogs	10 mL (0.338 fl oz) 20 - 30 ppm solution 2 x daily
Horses, cattle	30 mL (1.014 fl oz) 25 - 50 ppm solution 2 x daily

8.11 Hydrogen peroxide

Hydrogen peroxide consists of hydrogen and oxygen. The chemical formula is H_2O_2.

Hydrogen peroxide is used as a disinfectant in medicine.

Hydrogen peroxide like MMS and CDL/CDLplus is an oxidant. It can be effectively used to combat viruses and bacteria. For a long time it was an essential household and medicinal item. Hydrogen peroxide is used in medicine as an antiseptic for instance. It is also effective against fungi. It had been largely forgotten, though many people are now rediscovering it.

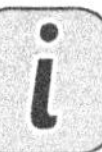

History of hydrogen peroxide

Hydrogen peroxide has been known for up to 200 years. In 1799, famed German naturalist and explorer Alexander von Humboldt (1769 - 1859) first synthesized a solution employing strong acids such as sulfuric acid diluted with water in Paris. Humboldt was astonished that the solute simply disintegrated when traces of metal, blood, or other bases were added: Oxygen was formed and only water remained. Hence the substance was designated "Oxygenated Water."

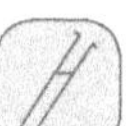

Treatment

A 35% solution of hydrogen peroxide for disinfection in the household: for such purposes as mouthwash, gargle and cleaning of contact lenses.

The hands can be thoroughly disinfected by washing them in a 3% solution.

Hydrogen peroxide is useful as a face cream to combat acne or skin blemishes.

In industry, 35% hydrogen peroxide solution is employed to clean returnable bottles, et cetera.

Hydrogen peroxide can be bought in drugstores in 3% and 6% solutions without prescription. It is applied mostly to clean wounds, which it does very effectively.

As regards animals its applications are many.

It is advisable to have hydrogen peroxide solution on hand in the home. When a child falls over, when one cuts a finger, when the dog hurts itself in the forest, or the cat comes home wounded from a night skirmish: Clean the wound with this solution. Infection can be avoided, healing encouraged. Needless to say, with larger wounds visit a doctor or veterinarian, and have the wound sewn or clamped where necessary.

8.12 Magnesium sulfate

Magnesium - a mineral that plays a significant role in relation to bones, nerve function, metabolism, muscles, and the cardiovascular system.

Magnesium is a mineral that the body does not produce and so must be obtained from nutrients. This has long been known in relation to humans and applies to animals as well. Just as with we humans, it plays a significant role for the health of animals' bones and various nerve functions. Nervous and/or stressed animals benefit from being provided with sufficient magnesium. This certainly applies to the metabolism, the muscles, and the cardiovascular system as well.

Many know magnesium as a laxative. In obstetrics MgSO4 (magnesium sulfate) is employed to relieve cramps for instance.

Magnesium is used to produce a highly saturated brine for flotation baths.

Magnesium sulfate is used to treat acute asthma attacks as well as acute heart attack. MgSO4 is used in flotation baths to produce a highly saturated brine allowing the body to stay afloat and not sink. These facilities are being researched in relation to sports medicine, treatment of burnout, and more.

8.13 MMS Gold

MMS Gold has nothing in common with MMS!

MMS Gold has nothing in common with Jim Humble's activated sodium chlorite MMS, more specifically the active agent chlorine dioxide with which it is often mistaken by users. This choice of name by the originator Leo Koehof is perhaps sly marketing trickery giving rise to much confusion with the public.

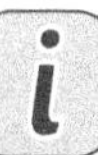

What is MMS Gold?

According to the manufacturer's data MMS Gold is a 10% mineral solution produced from a 20% basis solution of ionic minerals. The 10% mineral solution has the ability to purify and revitalize bacterially and chemically polluted water. The producer claims that with MMS Gold drops it would be possible to 100% cleanse every body of water in the world. In but a few hours all biologically dead lakes can be revived and brought back in balance so that the water is incontrovertibly fit to drink. Leo Koehof states this in his book "MMS Gold: The New Life Mineral" (MMS-Gold: Das neue Lebensmineral).

According to the manufacturer's information MMS Gold consists of the liquid extract that is obtained from black micaceous stone. This micaceous stone contains more than 60 minerals. The anorganic minerals are converted into ionic (liquid) minerals through a process of extraction employing sulfuric acid. These ionic minerals are negatively loaded and possess a surplus of electrons. Hence it can be said that the life minerals are electrolytic: when added to water a flow of current between negatively and positively loaded substances is generated. Poisons and faulty information are removed by means of an electrical load that breaks up water clusters (unstable molecular conjunction). A few drops of MMS Gold engender a natural circuit accompanied by a natural exchange of ions in water. Water is thus enriched with minerals and oxygen in a natural, primordial manner.

According to Leo Koehof MMS Gold contains important life minerals that are key to optimal cell function. "Vital" minerals boost the metabolism and therefore play a significant role relative to many bodily processes. Animals, which are more immediately connected to nature than humans, respond very well to treatment with natural substances.

MMS Gold contains many important minerals.

MMS Gold has even more positive attributes. Undesirable substances can be held and then purged from the body with MMS Gold, which also regulates the consumption of minerals.

MMS Gold:
a good nutritional
supplement

As with humans, nutrition is the linchpin for animals. The minerals contained in MMS Gold are not present in industrial animal feed. Animals lack access to the herbs that grow in mineral-rich soils. Hence it can be said that food causes our animals to be sick. By means of species-appropriate feeding and the balancing of absent substances with MMS Gold and moringa oleifera we can provide an excellent foundation for the health of our animals.

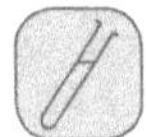

Treatment

Application according to Leo Koehof

Preventive:
Animals 50 kg plus (110.231 lb) 1 drop per 10 kg (22.046 lb) bodyweight in the drinking water
Animals 0 - 50 kg (110.231 lb) 2 - 5 drops

When sick:
Provide small animals with 2 drops in a little water 3 times daily; and large animals 5 drops with a little water 3 times daily.
This can be effectively administered by means of a syringe (without needle) directly into the mouth.

"The values that you pass on to others
are investments in your future
that will be abundantly repaid."

Jim Rohn

9 Nutrition

Species-appropriate nutrition is essential for healthier animal husbandry. I do not wish to stipulate what to provide, though I can perhaps encourage you to think about it. Even today the digestive tract and the organs of the dog and the wolf are hardly distinguishable from one another, little has changed over centuries of evolution. Likewise with other species such as cats and horses.

Species-appropriate animal husbandry is essential.

Horses have been domesticated for about 5000 years, but they are no different to the wild horse of that time. A horse normally spends 15 hours a day eating. It is on the move for over 15 hours each day. It instinctively runs away when in danger, and tolerates cold and heat very well.

Stable and open stalls:

Horses in a stall	Horses in the open stall / run
Feeding 16 %	Feeding 57 %
Standing 18 %	Standing 23 %
Lying 16 %	Lying 10 %
Being bored 50 %	Being bored 10 %

An open stall is a variant of stabling whereby a horse can day and night decide whether or not it wants to be out on the open pasture. What can be deduced from such a comparison? Being in a box/stall in no way corresponds to the natural behavior of our horses.

Stall versus open stall

They are barricaded in stalls and fed twice a day at most. A horse by nature eats for most of the day and is on the move nearly all day (as is indicated above). Does a horse really need muesli like a person does? Do we not all too often correlate the products, even the disorders, to humans, or more precisely industry? Is the incorrect nourishment of our animals the origin of various ailments such as diabetes, arthrosis (osteoarthritis), allergies, and so forth? Is all this not modeled on our human blueprint?

Extracts from an essay by Frau GallinAst: "Species-Appropriate Husbandry of Sports and Recreational Horses" (Artgerechte Haltung von Sport u. Freizeitpferden - EF Kinder und Jugendförderung eV www.electrofarming.de/cms/front_content.php?idcat=125, 25.01.2015):

"To violate the laws of nature can lead to suffering and unpredictable outcomes. The recent scandals in the food industry illustrate this yet again, unfortunately. Would we provide species-appropriate management for our farm animals, and we as consumers and producers finally put more value on ecological procedures and a healthier diet. Shortsighted, purely financially motivated strategies are not viable and harm the general public. We can be assured of high productivity in accordance with the existing genetic endowment of animals and plants without chemical and artificial expedients. We must be more attentive and analyze the situation more objectively for we all bear responsibility for our fellow beings.

... The new understanding concerns the improvement of feeding and care of our animals, especially the custody of sports and recreational horses.

The hope remains that all the customary commercial feed mixes are prepared with more rigor and with improved quality control.

Ingestion continues to be fundamental to the improvement of the health and vitality of our animals, the role of diet is central.

At the same time all changes must be conducted gradually. This applies to climate and the environment. If change is too abrupt then the digestion of nutriments is affected and many animals have no prospect of adjusting. If we do not attend to these external factors an imbalance in the organism will come to pass. Animals get sick or die sooner ..."

Ingestion is fundamental to the health of our animals.

This is just a short extract from the essay that considers conditions and physical activity further, and more. Thank you for the plain speaking.

The feed industry has positively exploded in the last fifty years. But what do our animals actually need? The cat eats mice; the only cereal that she might perchance eat is that which the mouse ate previously (often the cat does not eat the stomach). The dog is a hunter and gorger. He wolfs down as much meat as quickly as possible for typically he does not know when he will next bag some prey. Noodles, bread and other adjuncts are not to be found in nature to my knowledge. What he does find are plants and plant fiber to chew, these he consumes willingly. In my lectures on this topic I recommend BARF (Biologically Appropriate Raw Food), subsequently I am asked whether the meat should be cooked. I smile to myself and happily reply: "Recently I saw a wolf that had caught a hare light a campfire, and then barbecue it for hours."

"Recently I saw a wolf that had caught a hare light a campfire, and then barbecue it for hours." - Monika Rekelhof

Naturally our dogs and cats prefer the meat raw. The blood and water contained is their source of liquids. As I wrote at the beginning of the book, the protein content thus come by is also essential. Cooking destroys this, and for the animal it is relatively without value. In just the same way dogs and cats relish bones, chicken carcasses, chicken wings, and so forth. Now you will certainly be shocked and cry out: "Goodness me! Bones, they splinter and my animal might asphyxiate!" I would now like to ask you what our dog would do were it allowed to catch a chicken. Of course he would gobble it down hair and skin included, even better along with feathers and bones. Bones splinter when cooked. From drumsticks and the like you need generally have no fear. A genuine problem is the treatment of poultry with large amounts of antibiotics. Here too, each of us must decide for oneself. The same products are contained in industrial feed. I would prefer to buy species-appropriate and antibiotic-free

Cooking essentially destroys the protein contained in meat.

meat, but this is not currently realizable. At times one must compromise.

Dried feed overburdens cats' digestion and can lead to kidney disorders.

Cats, for instance, are desert animals and drink very little. They obtain fluids mostly from food. They are fed dried food however, drink too little, and as a result develop kidney problems with age. Food for thought, I think: Approximately six hours is required to digest raw meat whereas industrially manufactured feed, whether dried or canned, requires twelve. The long time it takes for digestion overloads the organism and the metabolism.

Dried feed no longer has nutritional value, is "dead."

Accordingly, dry food is to be avoided, and not for cats only. Even where quality raw materials are used, by heating to over 200 °C (392 °F) all the valuable raw substances such as amino acids, enzymes, and vitamins are destroyed. Dried food is "dead." The added substances are synthetically produced and are in no way equivalent to their natural counterparts. This is clear to see in the case of vitamin E that has a wide palette of subgroups only one of which can be synthetically manufactured.

More on this and other themes relevant to animal nutrition and animal health can be found in the book: "Veterinarians Can Damage the Health of Your Animal: New Paths in Therapy" (Tierärzte können die Gesundheit Ihres Tieres Gefährden: Neue Wege in der Therapie) by Dr. Jutta Ziegler.

To clone nature is not possible thank goodness, and I am thankful.

Many inevitably say: "Yes but, my dog, my cat, my horse is though ..." Naturally there is much more to say in regard to this theme, and there are always exceptions, but where should I begin and where should I end? For me what matters is to demonstrate how you might keep your animal healthy. There is so much information, and ideas that are new to you - the decision as to what you do with all this is entirely your own.

There are always very interesting reports and data to be found in the Internet. One can also gain some insight regards accrual and sales figures of firms.

Since when has pre-prepared food for animals been available? How were pets fed earlier on, and was this perhaps superior? For instance, one of our lecturers in alternative practice for animals (a veterinarian) proposed that the ailment hip dysplasia in dogs came into existence with the introduction of pre-prepared food. No scientific discourse is to be found unfortunately. And allergies likewise are dubbed fashion maladies. Why though has the incidence of these problems skyrocketed in the last years? The takeaway is: Nutrition plays a crucial role as concerns the health of humans and animals!

Hip dysplasia in dogs was first diagnosed with the introduction of dried food.

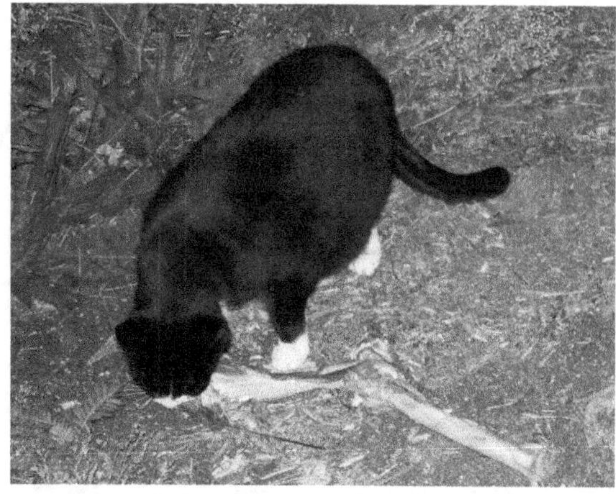

Our cat has nabbed a deer bone that was intended for the dogs, and, at a safe distance, is devouring it with gusto. Not all of it of course - that would have been too much for our Filou ...

Description practical example 1:

According to the veterinarian a client's dog was suffering from a food substance allergy for which a cortisone preparation was administered to relieve the symptoms of skin rash and itching.

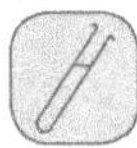

Treatment

We changed him over to BARF (Biologically Appropriate Raw Food). After about four weeks he needed no more cortisone. The symptoms turned to air and the fur grew back: a happy dog, and a happy owner.

Description practical example 2:

A client's dog suffered from diarrhea for years. All tests by the veterinarian brought negative results. According to the vet the dog was in good health.

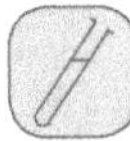

Treatment

The first step was to change the dog to a BARF diet. In a few days the diarrhea was gone, and so it remains. For the owner, who had a veritable odyssey with the dog behind her, this was a small miracle.

10

Conventional Methods of Treatment

10.1 Inoculation

A further, I find, very important and often controversial theme: With what and how often must I inoculate my animal, or must I inoculate at all?

In Europe only one vaccination is obligatory - this is the hydrophobia (rabies) vaccination, which currently must be repeated every three years. Studies by various universities here and abroad have however determined that inoculations employing current vaccines are still completely effective after nine years. Have we on one occasion taken the trouble to read the patient information leaflet regarding a vaccine? Usually we only see the syringe being removed, right? We blindly trust in the directives. Vaccines often contain heavy metals such as aluminum and mercury. Intuitively you will now counter that these substances can be expelled with MMS, but surely it is preferable better and more conducive to the health of our animals to steer clear of vaccines. Heavy metals cause illness; why then are thermometers with mercury no longer available? I am not saying do not inoculate - I find it important to be informed. However: Every sickness that the body has undergone facilitates the production of antibodies that enable the immune system to better resist bacteria, viruses, and the like. In order that our animals remain healthy take on the responsibility for your animal yourself, and do not hand responsibility over to others!

Vaccines contain heavy metals such as aluminum and mercury.

Veterinarians and proponents of immunization frequently endeavor to enlighten me as to how a non-vaccinated animal can jeopardize vaccinated animals. The question for me remains: How can my dog that is not vaccinated endanger a dog

Can non-vaccinated animals infect or endanger those that are vaccinated?

that is vaccinated? Should my dog be infected with Lyme disease due to a tick bite, it cannot to my knowledge infect a vaccinated dog - only a tick can do this. And with contagions such as rabies, my dog cannot infect a vaccinated dog if the inoculation serves its purpose.

On the theme of immunization I would like to quote from the book "Natural Medicine for Dogs" (Naturheilkunde für Hunde) by Dr. Wolfgang Becvar:

"... History has unequivocally demonstrated: 'Immunize' away one sickness and somewhere or other the next one materializes. So soon as the classic canine epidemics (distemper, HCC, leptospirosis) are 'immunized away', in at least our latitude, new epidemics that cannot quite be classified appear all-over. Think of canine parvovirus as engendered by a modified feline parvovirus. The conventional inoculation of indeed deadened (deaded), though undeveloped in terms of consciousness, pathogenic agents is not capable of extinguishing a 'sickness idea' whose trigger the various pathogens embody. The sick consciousness can only be emancipated by way of a consciousness raised to a higher power. The only means of countering communicable diseases long term is this: To transmute them to a higher plane. They thereby lose their negative influence on organic life and resolve themselves ...

... A little philosophy may at this juncture make plain that we should realize that nature's constituents - parasites are included after all - should be approached with farsightedness and insight. Accordingly, I see the only long-term effective prophylaxis of infections (besides adherence to the commensurate optimal living conditions) to be the dispensing of medications raised to a higher power (transformation rather than inoculation)."

"The only means of countering the communicable diseases long term is this: To transmute them to a higher plane."

Further to this theme, I discovered this very interesting article by Veterinarian Dr. med. vet. Danja Klüver (Source: p. 304)

"Inoculations represent a large part of the daily routine. The standard inoculation practice of up to now has of late been viewed critically by animal custodians, and rightly so. Have we veterinarians in the last years inoculated too often, an in combating too many sicknesses? Is a yearly inoculation really necessary? The recommendation on the package insert provided by the vaccine producer to refresh the vaccination in order that the immune system does not lose immunity issues from forty years ago.

Back then, preponderantly inactivated vaccines (even now leptospirosis or Lyme disease vaccines are deaded vaccines) that provided only short-lived immunity were in use. Today, largely live, attenuated vaccines that provide a very much longer period of immunity are employed.

In clinical trials (American Animal Hospital Association) vaccinated dogs indicated a seven-year if not lifelong immunity to pathogens when live, attenuated vaccines were administered. There are other German and English studies that have verified immunity-protection for nine years.

The immune system of dogs is demonstrably not worse than that of humans.

Current findings as to immunity-protection timespans allow for more flexibility when vaccinating dogs. Some vaccine producers (e.g., Intervet) have already extended their recommended interval to three years. Other manufacturers have requested an interval for rabies vaccines of three years only from the Paul Ehrlich Institute. That does not mean that these vaccines offer short-lived protection though. The statutory requirements for the recognition of new intervals concerning rabies, also for transnational traffic, are likewise founded on the alteration to the rabies regulation. When crossing borders with a dog

Recommendations regarding inoculation date back to the sixties when deaded vaccines were in use.

or puppy a veterinarian's note in the EU Vaccination Passport is standard and binding for customs officers.

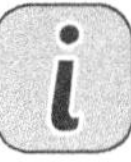

Intolerance to vaccines[1]

In principal every living being can suffer intolerance to or aftereffects from being vaccinated. There are acute reactions to inoculation and aftereffects that often do not appear for weeks or months, and therefore no connection with the vaccination is considered. The aftereffects can include diarrhea and vomiting, through to asthma problems, autoimmune illnesses, nerve inflammation, paralysis, meningitis, panniculitis (inflammation of the subcutaneous fatty tissue), vasculitis (inflammation of the blood vessels), injection-site-sarcoma (tumor on the site of the inoculation - relatively common with cats, very rare with dogs) anaphylactic shock (allergic reactions)!

Vaccination is also under suspicion for inducing allergies, immunity vulnerabilities, osteoarthritis and diabetes. The research in this domain is more than defective. Most research is concerned with the reaction of the body within no more than the initial two to three days.

The bottom line

Aftereffects are so good as not investigated.

For all these reasons I recommend vaccination to guard against life threatening sicknesses only. I would not immunize against trifling sicknesses, or those that arise very rarely. I would not inoculate to combat illnesses where the vaccine does not provide adequate protection."

---

[1] Dr. Danja Klüver, http://www.heiltierarzt.de/hunde-impfen/neue-impfpraxis-hundewelpen-schutzimpfungen.htm, 12. 06. 2015.

Note: This assertion comes from a veterinarian! Of course it is a question of priorities as to which inoculations are important and which are not. When going on holiday or when one lives close to a border, then it makes sense to vaccinate against rabies, as dogs when not immunized can be impounded by the police. Sometimes it is simply advisable to search out private accommodation for the duration of the holiday - again one decides for oneself and the animal.

10.2 Deworming

The theme "deworming" is a hot topic. Most veterinarians are of the opinion deworming should be undertaken four times a year. Many breeders chemically deworm whelps every two weeks as recommended by veterinarians. In the process of all these deworming procedures the intestinal flora is destroyed or at least forcefully attacked - the intestines thereby become increasingly vulnerable to worm infections. Resistance to such infections is already reduced during the puppy stage. It is seldom that a fecal sample is taken beforehand to establish whether deworming is even necessary. As a result of the many deworming processes in the puppy phase the immune system does not develop and the dog is later more susceptible to illness.

Many worm medicines impair the development of a healthy immune system in puppies.

A fecal analysis should be carried out if an attack of worms is suspected. It is also important to know which form of worm is involved: apt treatment is dependent upon this diagnostic analysis.

First response when worms are suspected: Fecal analysis

"Normal" worms can be effectively combated with MMS. Their little corpses can be seen in the stool after only one or two days. Other worms such as heartworms take longer to treat. It is crucial to match the dosage to the animal when treating worms with MMS. One can always put a few drops of MMS in the drinking water as a precaution.

Frau Dr. med. vet. Jutta Ziegler describes a good alternative to chemical deworming on her website www.drziegler.eu:

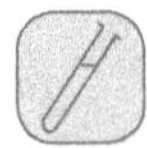

Treatment

"My alternative to chemical worm medication

- A day of fasting.
- Prepare a stock of ginger, garlic, and parsley; bring to the boil, and allow to cool. Give your animal 1 - 3 teaspoons directly to the mouth.
- Half an hour later administer 1 teaspoon to 2 tablespoons of castor oil according to the size of the animal - weakened and older animals should be given flax seed as a laxative.
- After another half hour give your animal a brew of buckwheat flour and elm bark or linseed."

There are very good plant-based deworming products available (cdVet Wurmovet). Tip for cat owners: Add herbal mixtures or the plant-based deworming medicine to a little natural yoghurt or sour cream (or something similar), stir in and offer this to the cat. This (there are many tricks) is among the most successful ways to outsmart a cat.

When combating worms it is important to purge with zeolite in the evening so that the dead worms do not produce gasses that might overload the liver and metabolism overnight.

Another possibility when tackling worms is diatomite (diatomaceous earth).

Diatomite is said to kill roundworm, tapeworms, whipworm, threadworms and hookworms within seven days when provided daily. It should however be administered for a further thirty days in order to eliminate the next generation as diatomite, like all other dewormers, does not reach the eggs. Important note: When lungworms attack, ninety days extra treatment is necessary, and with bandworms forty-five days. It is crucial when there is suspicion of infestation that the stool be analyzed to confirm whether worms are in fact present, and if so, what kind. Diatomite can be provided each day in the food to fortify the intestinal flora, though this is not beloved by cats. One should perhaps attempt to "sneak" the substance in: Try to mix a very little in to begin, and then increase the dose bit by bit. Definitely pay attention to the quality of the food in that the flea-killing substances available are not exactly appropriate.

Diatomite

Tip: A very effective pre-emptive measure for horses is to feed them diatomite with for instance walnut leaves as a side dish.

Dosage

I recommend 1 large teaspoon to 1 tablespoon of diatomite per day for dogs according to size.

10.3 Ticks and fleas

Spot-ons and collars contain a nervous system toxin that can have grave side effects.

With reference to "Vaccination" and "Deworming" it can be plainly said that by and large there are alternatives to chemical medication - it is not necessary to accept the first item on offer. The same is true for substances to counter ticks and fleas. These products, the "spotons" or "collars," familiar to almost everybody through advertising, contain a nervous system toxin that enter the animal's blood and can precipitate severe adverse reactions. I find it disturbing that I must handle such a product wearing rubber gloves and am warned that small children should avoid contact: Why then are these products still procured? They are obviously poisonous - not only for humans but our animals as well! They can lead to grievous brain damage.

Tip: Apply a little coconut oil to the dog's neck and to the base of the tail; add coconut flakes to food, and various herbal medicines as well.

Recently a dog owner related the following:
She had applied the spoton preparation to her dog as prescribed by her veterinarian. Shortly after, she was playing with and cuddling her dog when the following occurred: she sensed that one side of her face was paralyzed. This was due to the prescription! The dog owner herself told me that in future she would never again administer such a concoction to her dog!

Another very worthwhile substance against ticks and fleas is black cumin seed oil. A few drops in our darling's food will repel the pests.

In the course of treatment with DMSO no ticks appeared.

DMSO is also very effective. In the course of a treatment with DMSO it became evident that, as a side effect, there were no ticks apparent.

Should one of your animals have fleas, it can readily be powdered with diatomaceous earth (diatomite).

There are many other possibilities for protecting your animal from undesirable tenants. Search out a good veterinarian or therapist who offers alternatives to conventional medicine.

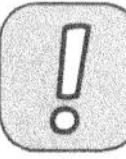

To ward off fleas, Satureja (savory) is cooked in water for several minutes, allowed to cool, strained, and filled in a spray container. Spray the animal with this. Fleas don't like it, keeping a wide berth.

This tip is from my dear friend Margret, and I pass it on to you gladly. Thank you!

11
Results of Scientific Research

Scientific research, studies, and patents are for many people very important. It is preferable to identify the inner voice and to trust in it. There has been much positive and much negative written respecting MMS and Chlorine Dioxide. The healing effect attendant to chlorine dioxide has by all accounts undergone much the same treatment as that which has befallen many new discoveries and inventions: It is first derided, then opposed, and after many years finally viewed as self-evidential.

Here I would like to refer you to the many positive personal accounts in Chapter 7. For me it is advantageous to have a substance such as MMS available for healing.

Apropos chlorine dioxide, there are scarcely any or only seldom published research findings, studies, and patents attesting to its healing properties. In the following pages I have written some things down which I ask you please, if you are interested, to research further for yourself. Here too, each of us is free to be inquisitive and to search the Internet!

11.1 Uganda Red Cross, Malaria study with MMS

The Water Reference Center in Uganda, an affiliate organization and representative of the Red Cross under the leadership of Klaas Proesmans (CEO Water Reference Center), organized a study of malaria in Uganda pertaining to the active agent chlorine dioxide (MMS). This project for which people with malaria symptoms were asked to sign on to was made public on radio. Hundreds of people submitted to a blood test as a result.

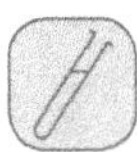

Treatment

Malaria was verified in 154 participants. The 154 persons were administered 18 drops of MMS for adults, 8 drops of MMS for children, and 2 drops of MMS for babies, one time. The MMS was activated with 35% citric acid and diluted in a ½ beaker water (babies received less water). After 24 hours the 154 people were again evaluated: By means of a blood test it was ascertained that already after one single treatment 150 of 154 participants were free of malaria, the remaining four malaria sufferers received a further single dose of the same amount as the previous day and then they too were well. This was corroborated with blood tests and recorded in written form.[1]

The bottom line of this study: 100 % success!

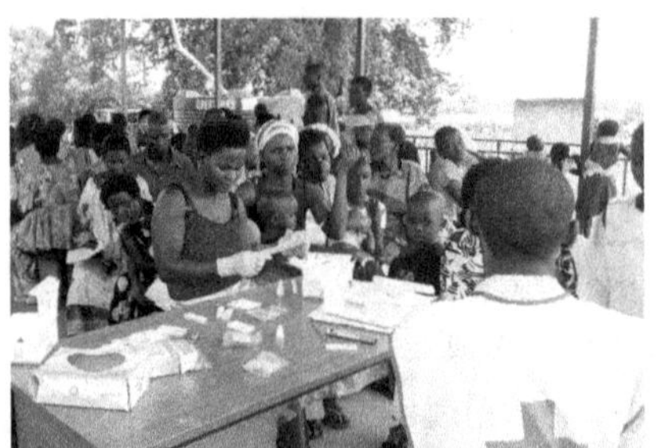

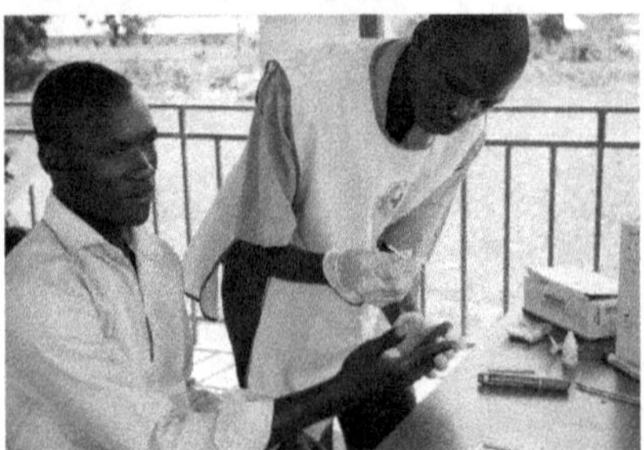

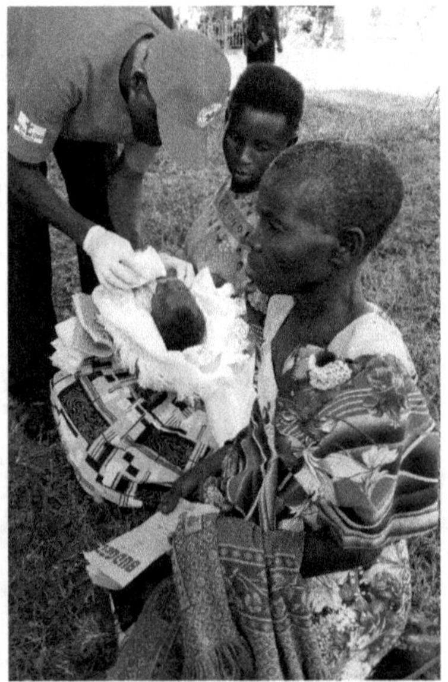

1 **Note concerning dosage:**
The dose was deliberately set high, as the dosage could not be progressively increased on organizational grounds. For most Europeans this dose is too high to begin with, and can lead to one to three days of queasiness and vomiting. The minimum dose possible should be administered initially, and, if time allows, increased slowly.

Unfortunately these studies were organized by the "lower echelons" more or less, which as the success with MMS became known resulted in several doctors being discharged, while the head of the study, who had himself clearly and forthrightly commented on the favorable outcomes on video, controverted his own study. As in the times of witch-hunts, chances are he was offered mercy should he disavow all that he had said.
In the course of this study 100% of the 154 instances of malaria was cured within only 48 hours!

In the film by Leo Koehof (German translation by Andreas Kalcker) everything is documented in word and image:
http://youtu.be/ZOO3U7PkXOw

Here is another film regarding this study:
http://www.youtube.com/watch?v=FvzuS9RqUl4

The Red Cross suppressed this video; the content was as a matter of fact contradicted afterwards even though the positive findings were documented loud and clear in sound and image. The video was made public by the Ugandan filmmaker who had been contracted by the Red Cross. All respect to this man for his moral courage!

The Red Cross wants to prevent the propagation of this video.

11.2 Chlorine dioxide studies by drinking water researchers confirm safety

Does taking MMS have negative implications for the organism? No! The 100 times concentration of ClO2 (chlorine dioxide), which is allowed and tolerated in our drinking water indicated no negative effects according to the governmental

100 times concentration is not dangerous

study by officers of the EPA (Environmental Protection Agency of the United States).

"Higher organisms are relatively unaffected by the intake of chlorine dioxide by swallowing. So for instance in a study on humans it was ascertained a one-time intake of 24 mg (0.000846 oz) chlorine dioxide in 1 L (33.814 fl oz) water, more specifically 2.5 mg (0.0000881 oz) chlorite in 500 mL (16.907 fl oz) of water, involving ten healthy men indicated no negative changes. This is a factor of ten, that is to say one hundred times the peak amount of 0.2 mg (0.00000705 oz) in 1 L (33.814 fl oz) for conditioning drinking water in Germany."

source: http://de.wikipedia.org/wiki/Chlordioxid, 28.01.2015.

11.3 Chlorine dioxide study WHO

**Chlorine dioxide study by the WHO:
No significant side effects**

"In a series of comprehensive studies involving human subject groups and chlorine dioxide as a drinking water conditioner groups of ten men were given a watery chlorine dioxide solution in an array of protocols (a series of increasing concentrations of up to approx. 0.34 mg/kg [0.749 mg lb] bodyweight over a 16 day period, and approx. 0.035 mg/kg [0.771 mg lb] bodyweight every third day for 12 weeks or approx. 3.6 x 10.5 mg [0.000370 oz] aqueous chlorine dioxide solution per kg [2.204 lb] bodyweight each day for 12 weeks)."
(Lubbers et al., 1982, 1984; Lubbers & Bianchine, 1984)

The observations comprise physical analysis (blood pressure, breathing rate, pulse, mouth temperature and electrocardiogram/ECG), comprehensive hemal biochemistry, hematology, and urine analysis, as well as subjective appreciation of flavor. **There were no significant side effects that could be detected according to the documented parameters.**

source: http://www.who.int/ipcs/publications/cicad/en/cicad37.pdf, 17.01.2015.

11.3.1 Death as a side effect

As can be ascertained from the ensuing figures (e.g., cancer): officially, more people die worldwide due to adverse reactions to conventional medicines. To this day not a single death resulting from being treated with MMS has been scientifically verified.

Death as a side effect: Conventional medicine versus MMS

You can gain an overview as well as numbers, facts, and interconnections regarding this for yourself in the Internet.

Almost 800,000 die yearly world-wide due to orthodox medical treatment.

Place 1: Deaths due to conventional medical activity (iatrogenic illness)
783,936 deaths yearly worldwide

Place 2: Heart Circulatory illness
699,697 deaths yearly worldwide

Place 3: Cancer
553,251 deaths yearly worldwide

Source: DEATH BY MEDICINE, 12 /2003
Gary Null PhD, Carolyn Dean MD ND, Martin Feldman MD,
Debora Rasio MD, Dorothy Smith PhD;
http://www.second-opinions.co.uk/deathbymedicine.pdf, 17. 01. 2015.

Aspirin and acetaminophen (paracetamol) bring about many deaths each year! The following appears on the expert portal for natural medicine for instance: An overdose of paracetamol can, according to Professor Kay Brune of the University of Erlangen, cause liver damage and even lead to liver failure. Quote: "We have a medication on the market which even with a small overdose is deadly. And it is not a pretty death, it drags on over a number of days." Similarly, pharmaceutical experts warn explicitly of aspirin - it contains the active agent acetylsalicylic acid (ASS) that is recommended for only those affected by grave cardiac and circulatory problems. Aspirin is recommended for heart problems only, how should I interpret this?

Place X: MMS

In the course of 25 years there have been no verified deaths. From infectious disease of all kinds to malaria, cancer, and autism chlorine dioxide (MMS) could bring about many recoveries.

The medical treatments of orthodox medicine often focus not on healing the sickness, but relief from a single symptom. When one suffers from high blood pressure for instance, one is prescribed medicine - life long. The blood pressure never normalizes long term. To counter the adverse effects that arise due to the medication more tablets are prescribed - life long. Billions are generated by means of this endless cycle. The damage to people attributable to this treatment of symptoms is immense. As per the statistics more people die of side effects of medicines than from cancer.

Naturopath Dr. med. Helmut Wagner reports in the expert portal "Naturopath" (12 / 90):

> *"In the course of my activities spanning sixty years as a doctor I experienced the coming and going of thousands of medicines such as Atophan for rheumatism and Pyramidon as a painkiller. They were prescribed the world over for years until they were proven to poison the liver and blood, and were prohibited. Thalidomide, considered*

to be an innocuous sedative, engendered hideous deformities in children of unsuspecting mothers. Butazolidin was for decades considered to be the best rheumatic medicine, selling more than180 million tablets until German television reported in December 1983 of more than a thousand deaths as a result of damage to the blood-building organs in England alone. That this medicine was prescribed worldwide for over thirty years is an example of how long it takes to acknowledge even deadly side effects. Just in the United States there have been approximately 140,000 deaths caused by medication registered in the last years - certainly but a fraction of the actual incidence."

According to Federal Public Health Office statistics there are some 24,000 pharmaceuticals whose therapeutic efficacy is unverified on the German market. Included are medicines for the treatment of blood circulatory and venous disorders, rheumatism, neuralgia, as well as mucolytic agents. That the health insurers must cover the costs all the same is due to a statuary period of grace for these so-called "grandfathered" (antiquated) medicines.

Germany: 24,000 pharmaceuticals whose therapeutic efficacy is unverified

(Source: AOK Stuttgart, member information 4/98)

Statistics furnished by the "Vaccine Adverse Events Reporting System" suggest that in the past 20 years up to 145,000 children have died as a result of this polyvalent vaccine procedure in the USA. Few parents are aware of this shocking figure. (VAERS - a program for the reporting of undesirable effects of vaccines.)

USA: 145,000 children have died as a result of multiplex vaccines in the past 20 years

"70 % of all medicines prescribed by pediatricians are administered more or less blind as no scientific data is available."
(Ernst Singer, Chair of the Ethics Commission
of the Medical University, Vienna,
http://www.intelligenzdeslebens.de/ seite19.htmL)

Hence, not only the side effects are alarming, the healing properties of all medications are in question. According to information from the numerous psychosomatic clinics (orthodox medicine) in Germany only around 5% of allergy cases can be cured. The success rate for other psychosomatic illnesses is little higher. Approximately 75% of all cases of sickness are classified as psychosomatic.

"... the pharmaceutical industry does not want us to educate and inform young doctors ..."

"Doctors do their best, but they do not receive all-encompassing, unabridged instruction ... The pharmaceutical industry does not want us to teach and inform young doctors ways one can heal oneself.
(Prof. Dr. Bruce Lipton, Cell Biologist, following 20 years teaching at a medical university,
http://www.intelligenzdeslebens.de/seite19.htmL)

In actuality the general public has already adopted this inference as regards orthodox medicine:

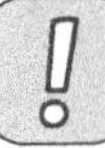

**"A cold lasts a week without medicine, and seven days with."
Most of us can endorse this contention on the basis of personal experience.**

The rate of recovery with orthodox or scientifically acknowledged therapeutic options appears to be very low. One can only first speak of healing when a symptom has vanished long term, without further treatment or medication being required.

11.3.2 ARD News

ARD report about malaria

In October 2013 the ARD Tagesschau (Daily News) broadcast a segment regarding malaria, the standpoint being that there is still no effective remedy for the disease.
http://www.youtube.com/watch?v=FvzuS9RqUl4, 17.01.2015.

When a storm of viewer indignation broke, drawing attention to MMS, the Tagesschau invited Prof. Jürgen May of Bernhard-NochtInstitute for Tropical Medicine to appear the following day.

He reiterated that there is no effective remedy for malaria, and as for MMS, there is no evidence that it works. He argued further that trials with MMS are not acceptable on ethical grounds!

How is this to be understood? Normally one expects that a talk show will present perspectives for and against. In this case there was only the against. Does this not give rise to questions? Why is not one person who has been helped by the medicine invited onto such programs? Why no mention of the studies (which, as I have since learned were proffered to the broadcaster - submitted in fact) wherein it is demonstrated that no pathogenic agent is resistant to chlorine dioxide? And that chlorine dioxide is an oxidant and accordingly a natural occurrence in the body; and that the human organism can deal with oxidation?

No objectivity in regard to MMS in the media

Another open question: What is unethical about this research? Is it somehow ethical to allow people to die of malaria? Is it ethical to administer noxious antibiotics that provide diminishing benefits to animals and humans? It has long been acknowledged that pathogens develop resistance to antibiotics. Is it ethical to ignore a study such as that by the Red Cross, to backtrack, and thereby hazard many people dying of malaria? Is it ethical to kill people by the thousands due to the side effects of

The "morality" of the media

common medications? Is it ethical for the WHO to deploy untested medications against Ebola where neither effectiveness nor the side effects have been established?

11.3.3 Ebola

Ebola is to this day officially not curable.

Ebola is a viral illness that can give rise to extreme fever and bleeding. The virus is transferred person to person via bodily fluids. The incubation period is two to twenty-one days. The first known Ebola epidemic flared up 1976 in Africa in the former Zaire. There is currently no effective conventional medical treatment by means of medication or vaccination.

As regards the current problematic with Ebola Spiegel online/ Gesundheit/Health 12.08.2014 stated: "WHO holds unproven medication to be justifiable!"

Effectiveness and side effects are uncertain.

From the Spiegel article:

> *"Doctors and aid workers in West Africa are still largely helpless: They have no medication, neither vaccine nor medicine, with which to combat the raging Ebola epidemic. Presently, only precautionary measures, travel restrictions, and the quarantine of patients are effective preventing further spread of the deadly disease.*
>
> *There are though a number of scientific advances in development of serums and therapies to fight Ebola. The problem: These substances are still officially in the test stage for animals. Merely a handful of patients, among them two US missionaries and a Spanish clergyman, have been administered doses of the unauthorized antibody cocktail in clinical trials. It is expected that existing supplies of the serum will be dispatched to Liberia.*

The application of such a medicine places experts in a dilemma: Which patients ought receive the medication? And what are the risks involved?

The World Health Organization (WHO) has now reached a decision and on Tuesday issued a statement in Geneva following consultations with medical ethicists: The deployment of the unauthorized medication in West Africa is justifiable given the dimensions of the epidemic according to an announcement by the WHO. 'The panel of experts arrived at a consensus that it is ethical given the extraordinary circumstances of this outbreak plus the compliance with specific stipulations to dispense untested substances with yet unknown side effects as a potential therapy or as prophylactic treatment.'"

Everything is "ethically sustainable" except for MMS.

Consider this: The inoculations subsidized by Bill Gates are 30% efficacious and can cause paralysis and more: is ethics accordingly not a problem?

11.3.4 Study chlorine dioxide and mosquito bites

Further evidence of the effectiveness of chlorine dioxide is provided by the Japanese Hiroyuki Matsuoka, Norio Ogata and Takashi Shibata: They documented, patented and made public its efficacy in 2011.
(See: http://docdroid.net/dg8x, 03.03.2015.)

This study determined that many millions of people in the world suffer and many serious diseases are transmitted by mosquito bites. The conclusions of this study ought to have caused a tsunami around the globe, but see for yourself.

The innovators named above conducted exhaustive tests aimed at preventing malaria infection at the initial stage.

The outcome was that an aqueous solution of chlorine dioxide on the skin forestalls mosquito bites.

The results of the study show:
By simply spraying a chlorine dioxide solution on the skin the amount of mosquito bites is reduced from 54.5% to 7.7%!

This signifies that millions of diseases, millions of deaths, incapacitation of millions of people due to epidemics in economically depressed lands could be counteracted were MMS in spray-form legally available to all!

11.3.5 The Story of Dr. Kurt-Wilhelm Stahl

Healing Wounds in Hell

The Freiburg medical practitioner Kurt-Wilhelm Stahl has for six years travelled through Afghan war zones providing medical assistance to the most needy (http://www.badischezeitung. de/ausland1/zumwundenheilenindiehoelle4219501.htmL).

A short extract from the article cited above:

Every fourth Afghan suffers from skin leishmaniosis.

"… There is suffering aplenty in Afghanistan. Every fourth Afghan suffers from skin leishmaniosis. Sand flies transmit the leishmania parasite that settles in the skin. Those infected do not die, but economic death looms. The wounds that stay open for years leave scars and mutilation behind. The victims are shunned. There are medications to alleviate this misery, but they are barely acknowledged."

Stahl implicates the pharmaceutical companies. The large drug companies neglect researching new medications designed to thwart tropical diseases as there is no money to be made from poor patients. Neglected sickness leads to neglected people. Stahl speaks loud on this theme:

Continual growth = cancer

> *"I hate this competitive thinking. A society where profit maximization dominates in every sphere of life is a society dying. We medical practitioners know only one term for permanent growth: Cancer."*

Non-governmental organizations such as the association "Waisenmedizin"(Orphan Medicine) founded by Stahl seek to counteract this predisposition. Together with Afghan colleagues from the German Medical Service in Kabul and the Leishmaniosis Laboratory in Germany Stahl has developed a new therapy costing 15 cents per patient daily. The wounds are treated with an antiseptic solution of Sodium Chlorosum. The scars are scarcely visible.

Three thousand patients have already been healed with this method at the Masav-i-Scharif hospital in the last year.

3000 patients in Masav-i-Scharif healed with sodium chlorite.

Sodium chlorosum is a pharmaceutical sodium chlorite; its antiseptic and tissue regenerating properties have already been confirmed. It is deployed against cutaneous leishmaniosis in emerging nations especially, as medicines are too expensive in these countries.

Yet again certain procedures are not clear to me. Where does the difference lie as regards pharmaceutical sodium chlorite and MMS? This pharmaceutical too is only approved for disinfecting water! MMS is sodium chlorite, just like sodium chlorosum. MMS is "demonized" and there are attempts to outlaw it, and then I read about this doctor and do not believe my eyes when I view the list of sponsors of his association.

His treatment with sodium chlorosum is supported by essentially the same organizations (including the WHO!) that simultaneously ban or ignore MMS. Many questions arise for me in this regard.

Sponsorship list of Waisenmedizin e.V. (Orphan Medicine), founded by Dr. Kurt W. Stahl:

Sponsors and Partners of WM e. V. - PACEM in 2008 and 2009

1. The World Health Organization (WHO)
2. The German Federal Ministry for Foreign Affairs (AA)
3. The German Embassy in Kabul, Afghanistan
4. The German Federal Ministry for Education and Research (BMBF)
5. The German Federal Ministry of Cooperation (BMZ)
6. The German Academic Exchange Service (DAAD)
7. Caritas International
8. Pierre Fabre GmbH
9. B. Braun AG, Center of Excellence Sempach, Switzerland
10. University of Erlangen
11. University of Heidelberg
12. University of Freiburg
13. Hôpital Universitaire de Genève (HUG)
14. Jérémie Gent Consulting
15. Ticuna Apps
16. Institut Pasteur of Alger

This gets one thinking ...

Another interesting pharmaceutical employed in the dental sector is SOLUMIUM, a dental treatment and oral antiseptic.

An extract from the directions of use:

"INSTRUCTIONS FOR USE OF SOLUMIUM ®
DENTAL SOLUTIION 30 mL
Dental and oral hygiene antiseptic agent
What should you know about SOLUMIUM ® DENTAL Solution?
SOLUMIUM® is a yellow, aqueous solution - the color and chlorine-like smell derive from the high purity chlorine dioxide (ClO_2) contained. There are no other ingredients. The solution may freely come into contact with the teeth, the skin, and the mucous membrane, but avoid spilling the product on clothes as it may discolor them.

Chlorine dioxide effectively kills all pathogens including bacteria, fungi, protozoa, and viruses. At the same time it has no harmful effects on the human organism. Its application as a disinfectant for the skin and the mucous membrane has been hindered as it was not available in the pure and stable form required. SOLUMIUM® contains chlorine dioxide of high purity thanks to a new Hungarian discovery, the ClO_2 solution can be stored for an extended period. Another advantageous feature is that chlorine dioxide can penetrate the skin and mucous membrane several decimillimeters thus disinfecting more than just the surface.

Chlorine dioxide is volatile: close the cap securely immediately after use, the solution will thus remain effective for a long time. The fading of the color indicates depletion of the solution. A colorless solution is ineffective.

The volatility of chlorine dioxide has another advantage, as it evaporates leaving no residue following treatment.

SOLUMIUM® Solution contains 0.12% chlorine dioxide and 99.88% water."

Dental Medicine: Chlorine dioxide's efficacy and harmlessness

Chlorine dioxide leaves no residue.

This claim is noteworthy: **"At the same time it has no harmful effects on the human organism."**

12
Patents for Chlorine Dioxide

All the following patents have been heretofore listed in the book "CDS/MMS: Health is Possible" (CDS/MMS: Heilung ist möglich) by Andreas Kalcker. More patents can be found on p. 84.

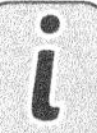

Patents

Patent US 2,70 1,781 from 08.02.1955 for the marketing of an antiseptic solution that contains Chlorine dioxide as the active ingredient for **general clinical usage.**

Patent US 4,03 5,483 from 12.07.1977 for the use of Sodium chlorite **as a non-poisonous antiseptic.** The text states that it would be useful in the treatment of burns and other wounds, and treating infections without inhibiting the natural regeneration process.

Patent 4,29 6,102 from 20.10.1981 concerning the marketing of a product to **combat amebic dysentery** in humans by means of oral administration of Chloroxiden. Patent granted to Felipe Lazo, Mexico City.

Patent US 4,31 7,814 from 02.03.1982, granted Felipe Lazo of Mexico for the commercialization of a medication for the **treatment of skin burns.**

Patent US 4,72 5,437 from 16.02.1988, loaned to the firm Oxo Chemie in Germany, in respect to a substance with the ingredient Chlorine dioxide, devised by Dr.Friedrich W. Kühne of Heidelberg and named "Oxoferin." **The firm was able to sell this for USD 45 million to an American concern, which renamed it "WF-10" thereby gaining authorization from the FDA.**

Patent US 4,73 7,307 from 02.04.1988 for the marketing of a product to combat **skin disorders** involving bacteria, fungi, and viruses.

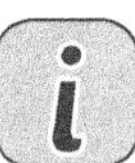

Continuation: Patents

Patent US 4,85 1,222 from 25.07.1989 issued to the firm Oxo for the marketing of a product containing Chlorine dioxide for the **regeneration of bone marrow.**

Patent US 5,01 9,402 from 28.05.1991 issued to the firm Alcide for the marketing of a product containing Chlorine dioxide for the **disinfection of blood and blood preservation.** It is primarily used in the branch of transfusion to avoid infections.

Patent US 5,25 2,343 from 12.10.1993 issued to the firm Alcide for the marketing of a product for prophylaxis and **treatment of bacterial infections,** particularly Mastitis, whereby 1000 ppm Chlorine dioxide is administered.

Patent 5,83 0,511 from 03.11.1998 for the marketing of a product also containing Sodium chlorite to **stimulate the immune system.** It was issued to the firm Bioxy, and is administered to animals as a food supplement. **It induces lowered mortality, reduced nitrogen excretion, decreased dependence on antibiotics and vaccines, and an improvement in the general health of animals by promoting a robust immune system.**

Patent 5,85 5,922 from 05.01.1999 issued the concern BioCide International for the marketing of a product containing Chlorine dioxide **that is used for the therapeutic treatment of poorly healing or non-scarring, chronic wounds, and other skin disorders.**

Patent 6,09 9,855 from 08.08.2000 for the commercialization of a product to **stimulate the immune system** issued to the firm Bioxy Inc. **This product is designed to improve animal health and the metabolization of food, reduce mortality, reduce dependence on antibiotics and vaccines, and improve the general health of animals by boosting immunity.**

13
The Rainbow Bridge

"The Point of no Return"

At times, when the soul of the animal has indeed decided to go, even MMS can unfortunately no longer help. It is very difficult to induce an animal to turn back once the decision has been arrived at. Typically, it all happens very quickly and we must say our goodbyes. Often this is not easy. In my practice I attempt to prepare the owner at the outset of treatment.

With some animals there is a fifty-fifty chance: In cooperation with the owner, all endeavors to turn the page to the positive are undertaken.

The animal decides how things will progress in any event. I respect this decision. Should the animal choose to go, I support the owner on this final journey, according to their wishes and as far as is doable.

To me, it is very important to show the living being respect - its decision too. A few thoughts and anecdotes relating to my work as an animal communicator follow.

13.1 When animals decide to depart, or greetings from Rainbowland

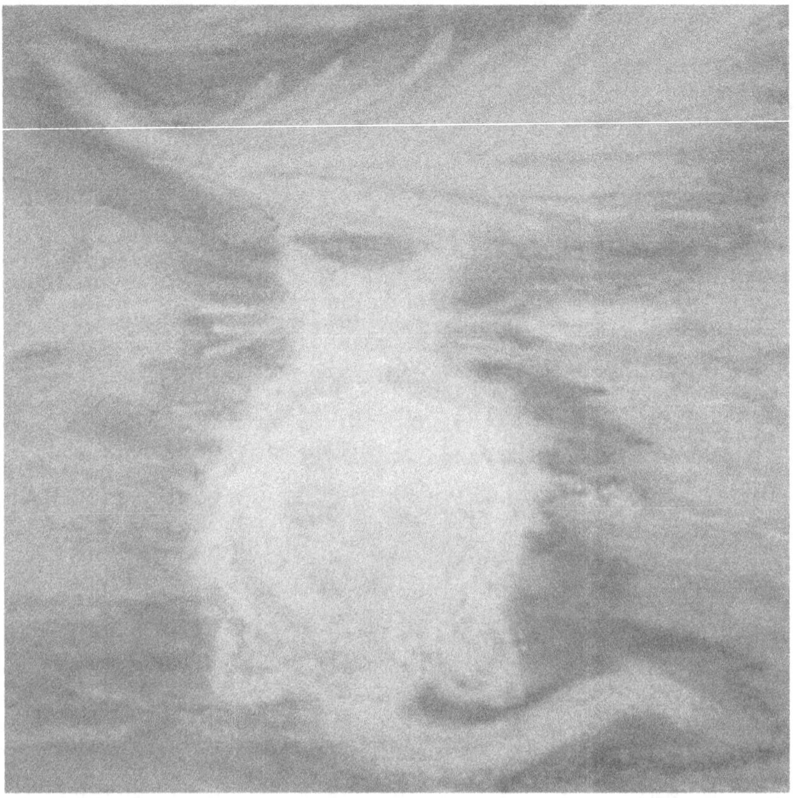

I frequently encounter death in the course of my conversations with animals.

I thereby sense peoples' fear and uncertainty. Question upon question: "Shall I have my dog put down?" "Is my cat suffering?" "Was my decision to put the animal to sleep correct?"

These are human questions arising from age-old fears.
Whence do these fears and this uncertainty derive?

Our parents, relations, or teachers took the decisions away from us as children. Our own intuitive and for us appropriate decisions were repeatedly corrected for being false.

We increasingly question what is right and what is wrong. We become ever less certain.

The press, television, politics, and religion have decisive influence. Meaning and value are scarcely examined for decades, or are instantly challenged. In this way our sense of accountability is undermined.

There are professions that we totally trust in, doctors and veterinarians for instance. That most people, including me, have not paid sufficient attention to illness and our bodies, and the bodies of our animals, it is simpler to put our trust in these persons in "white." When all is said and done they have studied this and on that account they know. We have learned this from childhood on.

Then day X comes.

All of the sudden, without warning, often utterly unprepared, we hear the veterinarian's diagnosis: "There is nothing left but to put the poor animal down."

Or: "Your dog is already fourteen years old and must undergo surgery. At this age, and because there is no chance of recovery anyway, perhaps it would be preferable to put it to sleep here and now."

But two examples that may come to pass. The owner now experiences fear, panic, and pain with full force.

All at once one must make such a grave decision?

What if one gives the wrong answer?

What if there is in fact another possibility?

Many questions race through the head in a matter of seconds. Then the acquired reliance on the veterinarian as savior clocks in and one gladly passes the determination on to he that surely ought know …

Our darling is consequently put to sleep, buried in the garden, or cremated.

In the days that follow:

Mostly we mourn alone. Family, friends, and acquaintances often greet our pain with amusement. After all it was just an animal. Why the theatricals? But for the most it was a beloved family member. Weeks, even years go by and we continue to agonize. Was it the correct decision? Was it the right point in time?

Only one thing is clear: One cannot go back in time.

On the basis of my conversations with animals I can reassure you: Animals live in the here and now … they do not question why. They do not dispute your decision and would certainly never reproach you.
A dog once asked me what would ensue if I now believed that it was indeed the wrong decision. The answer is of course: NOTHING!

When a cat decides today is the day, today I am going to sit on the street and let myself be run over, that is what it does. It also knows that it will with the next opportunity come back to earth in a different body if it so desires. Animals have no fear of a natural death. This fear resides in the heads of humans alone as has been cultivated over hundreds of years. Frequently our fear, panic and insecurity are transferred to our animals.

A good means of seeing how animals deal with oncoming death is to observe them in the wild. What does a wild dog, a wolf, a cat living wild do when it is sick or is old? It withdraws into a hollow or safe bush and patiently waits to die. It no longer eats or drinks and eventually goes to sleep. Our animals would also prefer to do this: They find a quiet spot, avoid food and drink, and wait.

But then there are humans. They panic, grab the poor animal, and rush off to the veterinarian. They believe something must be done. It is not acceptable to simply leave the animal be. We feel completely helpless. Our darling is suffering visibly. Who is it though that is suffering? We ourselves.

The animal has decided for itself. Our own decisions are so often put in question, why should we respect the decisions our animals make? Respect for one of God's creations?

Do we not wish that we too be treated with respect? Starting with our four-legged darlings we change our own life a little. Often it is not easy to take this step, but I can say from my own experience: It is a fine feeling and does one good.

And when actually should we commit to putting our animal to sleep?

Take this decision to heart and say farewell consciously. Your animal understands and is not angry with you. Look into the animal's eyes. Often they are already far away, their gaze turned inward. The animals are docile at the veterinarian as well. You have reached a decision - it was and is the right one!

It was not over for a young girl whose beloved cat died after running in front of a car. She reacted hysterically when the name of her cat was even mentioned. I showed her, with her mother's understanding, animal communication. The cat told the girl that she should no longer fear. It would nevertheless still creep into her bed each night and take care of her. The girl could see and feel how happy the cat was. She also saw an old woman with the cat and recognized her dead granny. To the girl's delight the cat also showed her a picture of a dog in whose body the cat would return to her. From then on the girl could speak of the cat without problem.

Each person that partakes in my courses in animal communication brings pictures of animals with which they wish to talk along. These pictures are then distributed on a table in center of the circle. Each of the participants searches out a photograph. In that photos of dead animals are among these, participants often receive such a photo. They prefer to hold these images covered up, or pass them to me. I hand them back and allow them to be passed around. I like to mix in photos of my dead animals without mentioning anything bar the names. Often, when they speak with the animals they are unbelieving yet fascinated. They are surprised how easy it can be to talk to dead animals. Talking about death and mourning thus becomes easier. Frequently, during a face-to-face conversation, comes the next question: "Can one also speak with dead persons?" There are people who can. Look for a medium you can trust with whom to have such a conversation.

At one of my animal communication seminars I handed a photograph of my dead tomcat to a participant. I would like to make known that this woman doubted herself and her ability to learn to communicate with animals. The tomcat repeatedly told her in animal-speak that he is a female and not a tom.

She looked at me disappointedly and believed that she would never learn animal communication. Smiling, I showed her a picture of my little cat Sheela. I then explained that this is the incarnation of my tomcat, and that the tom is now a female cat. She was speechless. Yes, at times it is not immediately clear what animals might want to tell us. That this woman locates strays and has no more problems with animal communication gratifies me.

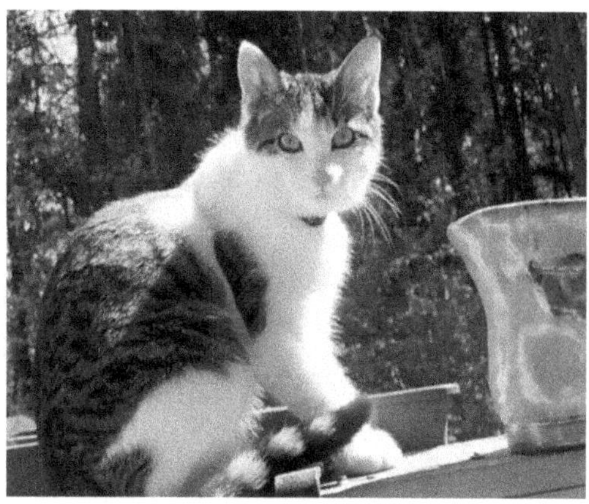

In the course of a conversation with an animal soul an image may be transmitted into my thoughts. I then paint this. The first picture came from my tom Schnaxl. He named it "Seelenpinsel" (Soul Brush). He prompted me to offer this opportunity to many others. They are not artful oil paintings. Frequently I produce the pictures with chalk. I serve, so to say, as a tool with which the animal souls paint. When the picture is complete very often I think, "What's all that mean?" To my surprise the owners understand exactly what the animal is trying to communicate.

While speaking with a cat I saw it sitting in a window. Later, I thought I would paint this. The picture: A woman is lying before the window a yellow blanket pulled up to the chin, and above her head lies a cat. OK, we'll see what the owners have to say: The couple looked at the picture for a moment, both shaking their heads. "That can't be possible!" they exclaimed. The woman explained that she had for some time practiced yoga and breathing in front of the window. Often she remained there relaxed still covered by the blanket. On such occasions the cat would bed down above her head as in the picture. Recently she had often thought to do these exercises again. Is there a sweeter invitation? Certainly none more loving.

It is wonderful work for which I am grateful each and every day. Frequently tears fall while I do this in my practice. They are seldom tears of sorrow, but mostly liberating. What could be more pleasing than to see your animal running joyfully thru a flowery meadow?

One day a tearful friend called me. Her beloved horse had died. I calmed her a little and promised to look out for the horse. The mare relayed a beautiful image: She was galloping with a stallion across a meadow in flower, a rainbow in the background. The other horse had a magnificent mane. I sent my friend the picture and told her of the other horse. She replied: "Yes, that was my mare's great love. The stallion had to return home to his stables a year ago. Lovesick, he refused his feed and died. We heard of this much later. The stallion, his soul rather, was with his beloved mare all year and now they are reunited in Rainbowland."

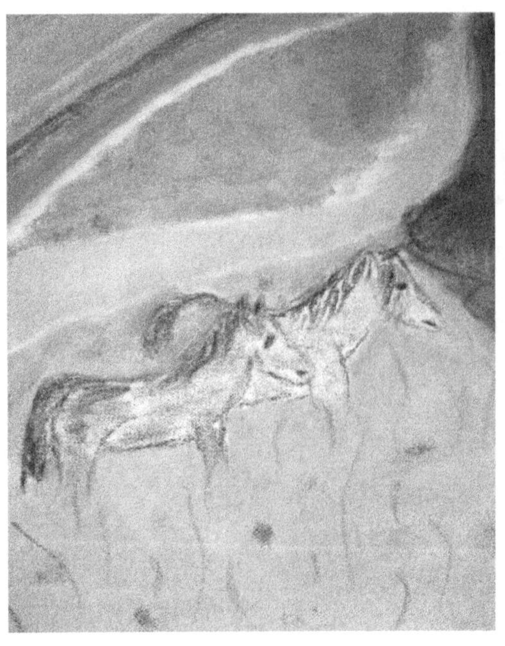

In some cases our animals seek to make us aware of something by their dying. For instance they wish to point out our fear of loss. Often our fear is to be no longer able to control something. Generally, when our cherished quadruped dies we have no control. We are wholly unprepared. We cannot and do not want to understand. We are often angry at our treasure.

Why now? Why couldn't she/he wait? Why am I left behind alone? These are questions concerning ourselves and our momentary circumstance.

The dog of an acquaintance died. She was able to make contact with him, yet she could not come to terms with the new situation. One day, without invitation, the dog stood before me in my mind's eye and relayed an image that showed a crouched woman enclosed in a rock girdled by bright yellow light. My spontaneous intuition was: When will she stand up and so shatter the rock entrapping her heart? When we met, I gave my acquaintance the picture. She looked at it, nodded, and then came the first release of tears. She was so thankful to her dog.

I find talking to souls to be such a wonderful gift. As often as not people suffer profound wounds and a deep scarring of the soul when they cannot let go of their pets that have died. In many instances I advise seeing a therapist. Whether to do so or not is your decision alone.

A principal for me in my practice is: I can suggest and explain something to someone, but to reach a decision and therefore act, to move, only they can do that. It is a matter of respect for all living things.

One word should be struck from one's vocabulary: MUST. Regardless which domain, private or professional, frequently it is: "you must this" or "you must that." I tell myself: "I must nothing. I may do it, or not." You can observe your own body for example, or your pet's, when you ever and again do what you actually do not want to do. A friend told me, for instance, she always gets back pain when she acts against her will.

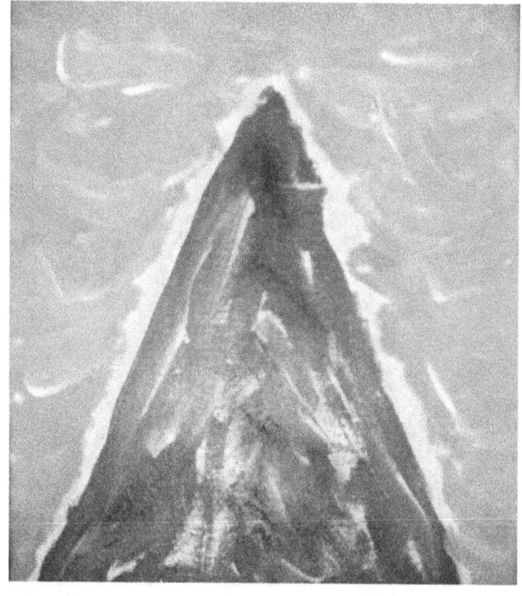

Back to our animals: Why does it weigh us down when we must put our animals to sleep? Have our senses told us "no" although we have allowed the veterinarian to sway us? By no means do I want to criticize your decision or engender doubt. Perhaps this is of help finding a new way of thinking and to climb off of the old thought merry-go-round. For all things, such as, the purchase of this book "MMS for Animals," or now, by reading it, you yourself arrive at the decision.

Life can be so beautiful.
A maxim by Charles Darwin:
"All that is against nature cannot long survive."

One day a woman came to me and asked for me to make contact with her dog that had died. He showed me his soul image mentally and I painted a path. This path was very rocky, trees were sawn down left and right, only stumps were to be seen. In the distance, behind a little curve, a yellowish light was evident. My interpretation was that the woman still had a rocky path ahead of her, but beyond the curve it was bright and good even though it was not yet apparent.

The woman looked at the picture and was very pleased.
"This is where I always walked my dog. I recognize and know where it is."

Two insights, both correct in their way: It is in the eye of the beholder. What does one wish to see, and then the viewpoint from which one sees. Of course from the outside I see things differently. If my customers so desire, I express my view. Here too, each decides for oneself.

One of my painted soul images shows a cat on a sailing boat. It seems everything is possible in Rainbowland. On one side is a cloud and yellow light. Anyway that is how the picture came to me. I took it to the customer. When she called to speak about the picture I was totally amazed at what she saw there. She said, just as with the cat, a stiff breeze was blowing in her face. I asked: "Which breeze?" I had no idea of what this could signify. The conversation continued. The picture was standing in the living room when I next visited her. I contemplated it for a while; then I could see the wind as well. I am again and again fascinated how it plays out. I cannot nor do I wish to explain it. One thing though: I am very grateful for this talent. In this way I too am learning to have a different attitude to death, the fear is developing more and more cracks and can its take leave. My tomcat Schnaxl was and is a great help. He indicated the gateway to animal souls and did away with my fear of it. The first step was when my tom Felix died and I was able to see beyond. At the time I was not yet so far as to appreciate the beauty there. I let my pain be, and that was good.

A friend asked me to speak with her dog that had died years earlier. She was already able to do so herself, but was afraid. I offered that we walk the path together. Frisky and full of joy it ran up to her. She was so happy to see it that she began to cry. I pointed out how well it was doing, and how delighted it was to see and finally talk with her. 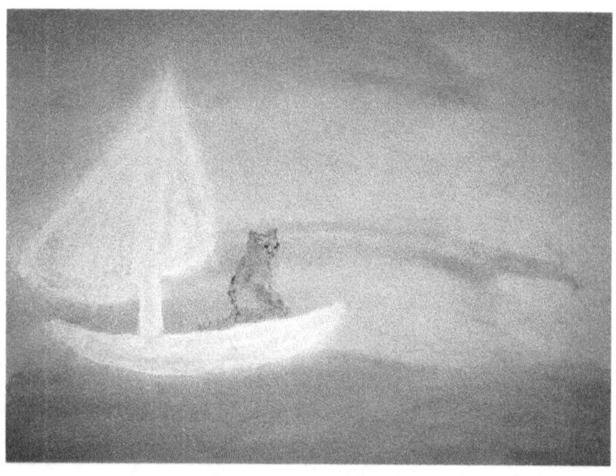 After a while it said it would return to her. Initially she would not recognize it for it would look quite different.

Yes, and so it came to pass: We had just worked through something together when our dog grandma Maggie became present as promised. When my friend saw the energy of the old German shepherd bitch a ball of light suddenly appeared. One could feel only love. Wonderful unconditional love. My

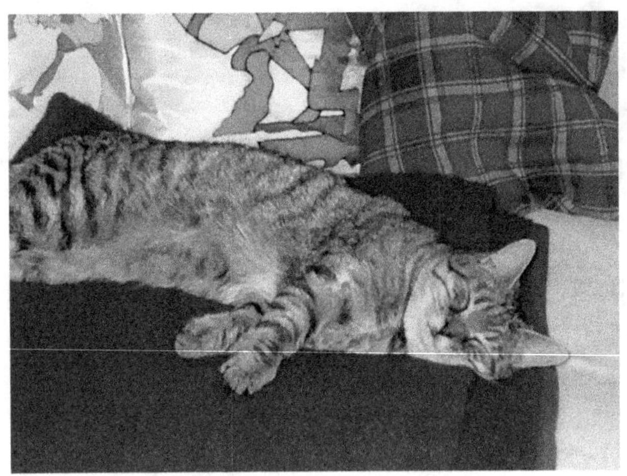

friend asked whether one of my cats had come, my first thought though was that it was her dog. She began to cry again, as it brought the feeling of unconditional love back as a gift. It then bid her farewell for an indefinite period. If she for some reason might need assistance she should call on her any time.

14

Animal Communication

The subject "Animal Communication" lies close to my heart. Many people still find the notion to be suspect. It is farfetched as dogs can only bark and cats meow, how can they tell us anything? Animal Communication transpires telepathically, necessitating a heart to heart connection.

"What does animal communication have to do with this book?" many would surely ask. Animal communication is for me a way to ascertain the cause of the current problem, no matter physical or psychological, to experience the origin, so to say, of the condition - a horse's loose stool can indicate many things for instance. When a horse conveys this as being the response to an alarming experience and I treat the psychological realm, I am soon able to realize a positive outcome.

Very often the animals suffer emotional problems. Being that they frequently come from animal welfare or an animal home the owners do not know what may have come to pass earlier in the animal's life. In such circumstances I can figure the situation out by means of animal communication. It is also helps with the administration of MMS as I can enhance this with other substances and tinctures.

What constantly astounds me is the immense knowledge animals possess. Often they identify substances of which I have never before heard, or read about. It is remarkable to discover when researching in my books that they are always one hundred percent applicable. With the aid of examples drawn from my experience I would like to spark your interest, and

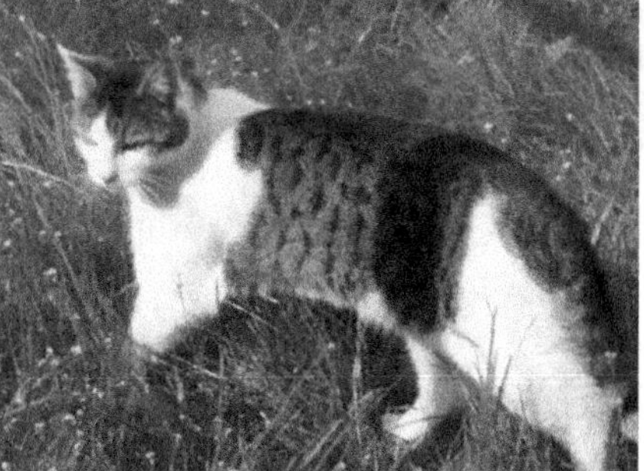

perhaps direct your attention to the wide array of possibilities proceeding from this kind of interaction.

14.1 What do animals wish to show humans?

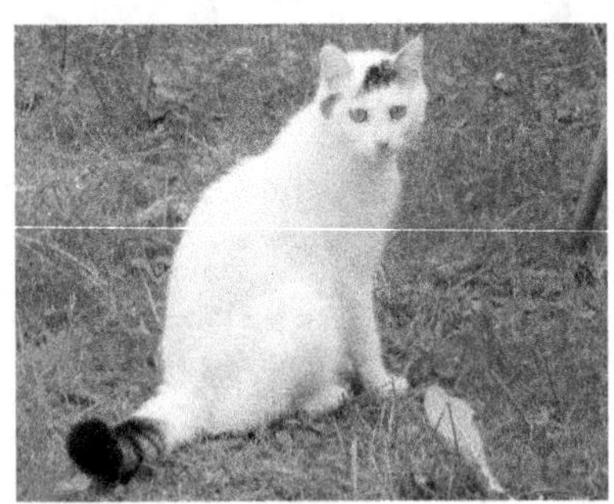

Humans and animals: coexistence arising from consideration and respect

Today I read a pleasing clause in the book "Anastasia - The Energy of Life" (Anastasia - Die Energie des Lebens).

"Question to God: *'What do you most desire?'*
Reply: *'Collective creativity and the ensuing joy experienced by all on viewing our achievements.'"*

This motivated me to write these lines. We'll see what I accomplish with the help of the animals. I hope it brings you and me pleasure!

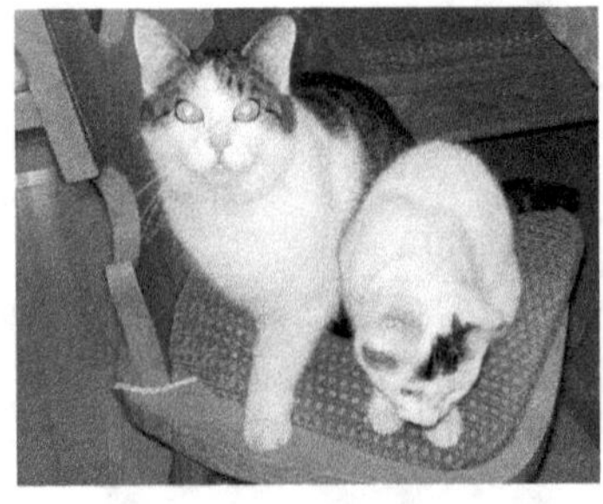

My little Sunshine is almost six months old. When I tell acquaintances that a second cat has come to me the question is usually: "How do they get on?" They get on very well of course. They are a great team and my Schnaxl has already taught her a great deal. They love to play with one another, and a lot.

Mostly, there are troubles on the arrival of a new cat in a home where one or more cats already live. When I relay that first I asked my tomcat whether Sunshine could come I am looked at quizzically, whereas for me this is but a matter of course.

What is it like when a new partner comes into the life of a person? A couple of weeks before Sunshine arrived a new partner came into my life, I informed my tomcat of this as well. Here too there were no problems.

I ask myself whether the fear of the new is a human trait? When we see a small cat and think "I'd like to take her with me," what as a rule happens in out thoughts? Questions arise such as: "Goodness, how will my cat at home react?" or "Will she defend her territory?"

Why is this so?

A nice thought for instance might be the following: One pictures the two cuddling and playing. This image is taken home in thought. One also retains the pleasant feeling that this thought has generated. I can imagine that the mood in the home would be harmonic from the start.

We ought pay more attention to our thinking at any rate.

My two cats provided a good example. When Sunshine took her first excursions out into the garden my tom looked out for her. I often thought to myself: "How do I teach the little one that living food such as a mouse has no place in the house?" It had worked out great with my Schnaxl. How would it be then with the little one? I pictured her playing with mice inside the house; since she could not enter and exit on her own it was not yet an issue. I was indeed mistaken. Schnaxl got involved by simply bringing a mouse in for her after a foray, and Sunshine had great fun with it. Subsequent to my initial incredulity, there were three occasions where I interceded by rescuing the mouse and taking it outside. It was necessary to have a number talks with the two. The old regime is again in place. Those two, they are certainly special!

One great fear I had was that one of my cats would bring a snake home. I have a pronounced aversion to these animals. Of course Sunshine fulfilled my "wish" one evening. It was both a shock and instructive. I will take more care as regards such thoughts in future.

Another theme also causes me great concern: Do we humans permit the animals with which we live to be animals or do we overly anthropomorphize them?

I live in a rural district. It is presently winter here. I frequently see horses in the paddocks while driving my car. I find it odd that many wear blankets. Why? A horse in fact endures the cold without a blanket. Supposedly the owner suffers from the cold easily.

Unfortunately, it has often to do with the "beauty aspect" only. By means of the cocooning the owner can avoid the not pretty springtime molting season.

My friend has a cat that is just a little stout. I have often been forced to smile when visiting. Now and then my friend goes out on the balcony to smoke. Missy happily accompanies her outside. When my friend has finally finished and is feeling cold she insists the cat come inside - she will most certainly freeze. I have made her aware that Missy is a cat and wears a natural fur coat. We laugh at that.

An acquaintance who has a number of cats contributed another example. Behind his house is a creek. He once told me of looking on with horror as his cats repeatedly drank the dirty creek water. He thought he would procure fresh spring water for the cats in particular, and for himself. He tendered this water to his darlings at various spots in the home. Cats though lap up dirty water from roof spouting and puddles.

Spring water is doubtless very good for humans, but for a cat?

I am often reminded that animals know instinctively what they do or don't need. They decide, with water too, which minerals they currently require. I must smile when I advise owners to try this or that substance out with their animal. The dismayed response: "My cat or my dog won't stomach that! It smells in extreme!"

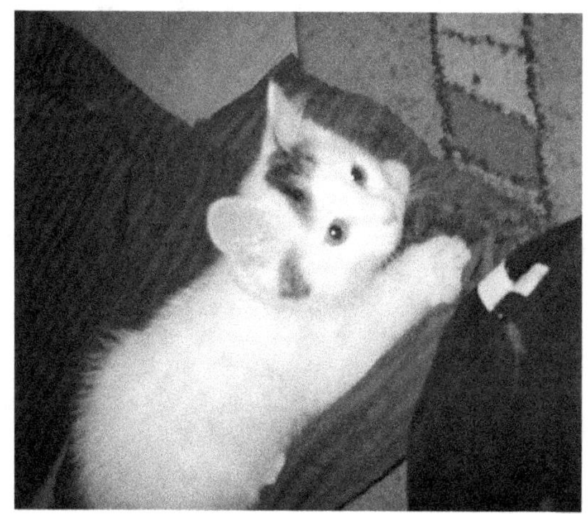

Another example from my friend: Her cat Missy ought take MMS, which, as you know, smells strongly of chlorine. My friend took these drops herself at one time and found them to be ghastly. As Missy is very particular about her food my friend doubted that Missy would accept the medicine. Well, surprise: Missy swallowed it without hesitation. On the second day she was most insistent, she sensed she needed it and pointed this out to her mistress categorically.

My friend began to wonder what it was the cat was telling her regarding her attitude to her own nutrition and medication. Concerning food, she is just as fastidious as her cat. I have heard similar things from vegetarians who attempt to convert their sweethearts to the same attitudes as their own as concerns meat. Naturally, it does not work, or the animal develops signs of deficiencies.

Relative to this theme, here is a lovely poem by my friend Algiz who is also vegetarian:

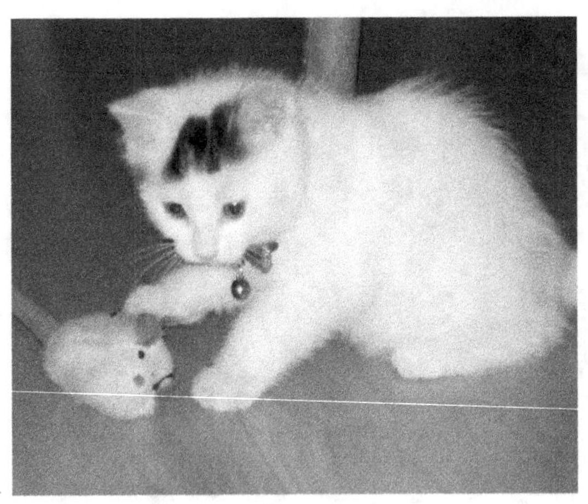

Cat Dream

Plaintive mews the cat from where she lies
Her dinner she would best decline.
Would rather gorge on sausage
But mummy most regrettably
Eats only fruit and vegetable
And some grizzly herbs found in meadows.
So all that remains is for the cat to dream
Of a delectable sausage tree.

Algiz

The "babysitter" of my two cats is now twelve. Sometimes she comes to tell me that my tom has caught a bird or a mouse. She is distraught and downright angry each time. I try to explain that this is absolutely normal. Cats are by nature predators. I am also convinced that those animals are reconciled with being fare for the tomcat. This cheers her. She loves animals, and would save each and every one of them.

Another hot topic is reincarnation, and the death preceding.

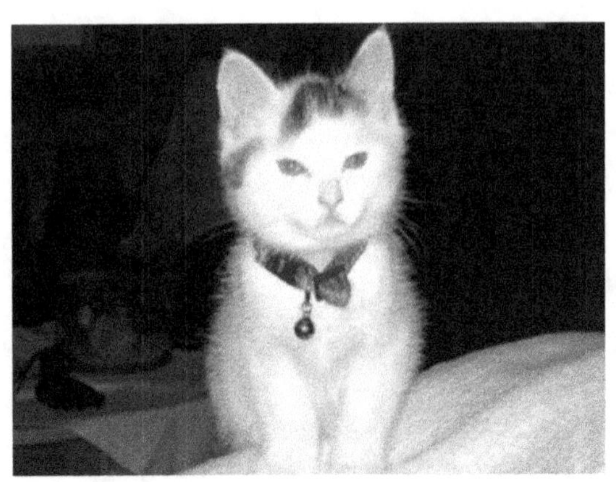

My Sunshine wanted to tell me something one evening. I asked her: "What do you want to tell me?" At that she put on a performance. First she ran about like a crazy thing, jumped onto the windowsill, then fell down. I ran over to her to check, you would have thought she was dead. Looking closer, I could see she was moving. The movements were peculiar though. Her hind was lame. I gathered myself and reflected. A thought came to me and I asked: "Are you Batzi?" She answered with a little "Yes." Batzi was my son's favorite Degodi lark. It fell out the window and was paralyzed at the hip. Despite the hindrance it lived a while longer and experienced the joys of being a father with a new, young and pregnant mate. I was very pleased by his decision to become incarnate through my Sunshine and to return. Together they resolved to be my teacher.

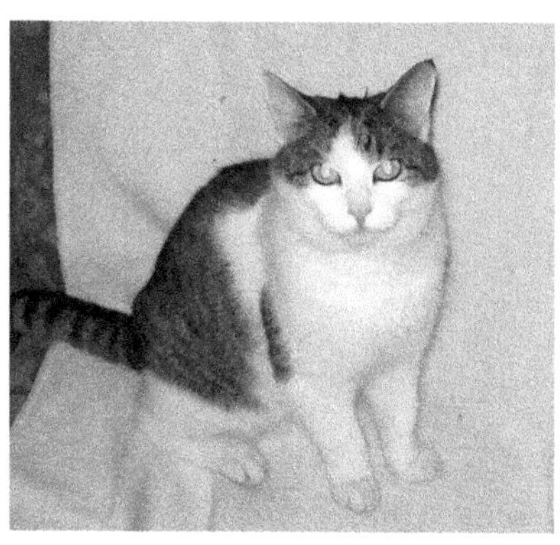

My sweet Schnaxl did not come home one day. It was spring and I supposed he was outside running about with his buddies. After two days I asked him: "Where are you?" To which he answered that he was underway. Well yes, I thought, I already gathered that. A couple of days later he showed me a fox and a hollow. I thought to myself, good, he had a hollow as a shelter to sleep in. I was very wrong!

A few more days and he showed me his body being consumed by maggots and other creatures. It was now painfully clear that a fox had nabbed him and hidden him as booty in its lair.

At the same point in time the little one indicated that he was doing well and relayed that he would soon come back to me.

In addition, he sent me a beautiful soul picture and suggested I allow other people who were obliged to say goodbye to their beloved animals to see this.

I have had the opportunity to do this many times and it is always a wonderful experience. Thank you to the animals that grant me so much love and enable me to feel this love.

My Sunshine became a mama. A number of weeks prior to delivery she made known that four souls were waiting to be embodied. Soon after I noticed she was pregnant. It was the

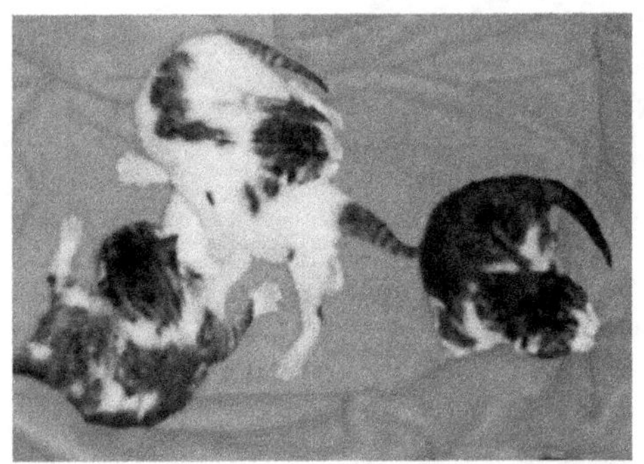

beginning of exciting times. When would these little worms commence making their way in the world?

Sunshine did wonderfully. She brought the babes to the world alone, and is a fantastic mum.

My tom Schnaxl became incarnate as the little Sheela; Timi, a little tomcat, is a friend's dog. It is simply beautiful to experience this all.

Often I am asked whether I am afraid when I make a connection with an animal spirit. I can only say no. It is so gratifying, and I experience so much love and appreciation.

A little tomcat was baptized Kosmo. He is really quite special. "How does one arrive at a name like that for a cat?" I am often asked this, or: "Your cats have funny names!"

My, and many other, animals are simply asked what their name is. Little Kosmo explained he came out of the cosmos, that's why. Another cat confidently told her owner that her name is Cleopatra. The owner asked whether she might call her Cleo which both found to be acceptable. I heard yesterday of a street dog in Spain who informed his chosen owner that its name is Vishnu.

I am always delighted when I can demonstrate animal communication, when I see the looks of amazement and then hear: "It actually works, and it's so simple!"

Recently I instructed a boy. He was beside himself and said: "I saw the cat clearly; she was asleep!" A little later he came from outside with the cat in his arms. He was very excited and cried out to his mother: "Look mummy, I found her exactly where I expected, and she was sleeping too!" He was very happy. I smiled and asked: "You did not believe it, and now you have made certain that it is so!" "Of course," he said grinning. "It's cool. I'll try it out more often!"

A reaction like this certainly pleases me enormously.

Something that deeply concerns me is the faith people have in doctors and

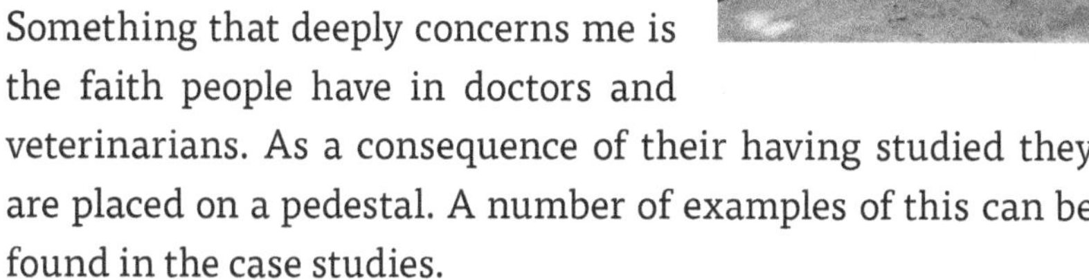

veterinarians. As a consequence of their having studied they are placed on a pedestal. A number of examples of this can be found in the case studies.

A friend and animal owner asked for my help. Her friend was in tears and her bitch totally distraught. I drove there right away. When I enquired what the actual problem might be the owner told me they had been to the veterinarian. The diagnosis was a mammary carcinoma and a lymphatic gland tumor. I could not confirm this with the initial tests though. The owner assured me the vet was one hundred percent certain.

What then is "one hundred percent"? An appointment to operate at the clinic was arranged for that same week. I guaranteed that the dog would come home without being operated upon whereby I was met with total disbelief.

Smiling, I arranged with the dog to show them all how one hundred percent really looks.

What to say? The operation did not take place. The veterinarian could not confirm the findings. Jubilant, they returned home.

I could report further, but I only wish to ask that diagnoses from veterinarians be thought through, and perhaps reviewed.

At one of my workshops I came upon a new and interesting theme.

What do animals feel when people separate? How do they cope with the new situation?

A woman separated from her husband. The dog resided with the man the understanding being that it belonged to him. (On the theme of "ownership" please read below.)

Due to the separation the self-esteem of this woman was nil. She felt she had forsaken the dog and thus felt guilty. She believed the dog must be in poor shape as it was alone all day while the husband was at work. Each day she went over to the husband's place in order to take the dog for a walk.

When she learned how to communicate with the dog a smile magically appeared on her face. The dog was in fact content with the situation. The husband needed him more, and she came by anyway. Everything was just fine.

Maybe it is our hurt pride or ego that has us think this way.

And now to another fascinating topic: Ownership.

May we, can we, own an animal?

I am aware that our animals have decided for themselves to spend some time with us and to live with us.

And what then if an animal resolves to live elsewhere? Do we respect this decision, or do we force the animal to return to us?

I think it is mostly the latter. We believe we have this right and behave accordingly.

For the most part, the same happens with kittens and puppies. They arrive in the world: What then? As for "my babies," people came by and asked to have one. I explained that it is not for me to decide, rather the babies themselves. They will choose their place of dwelling.

That is how it panned out. Mika chose her home, a very agreeable place abundant in meadows, forests and fields. She was a loner from the start, and could live this out in her new home.

The little lady sat herself uninvited in the cat-box half an hour ahead of departure and waited there.

There was no wailing and lamenting. She is very happy with her home.

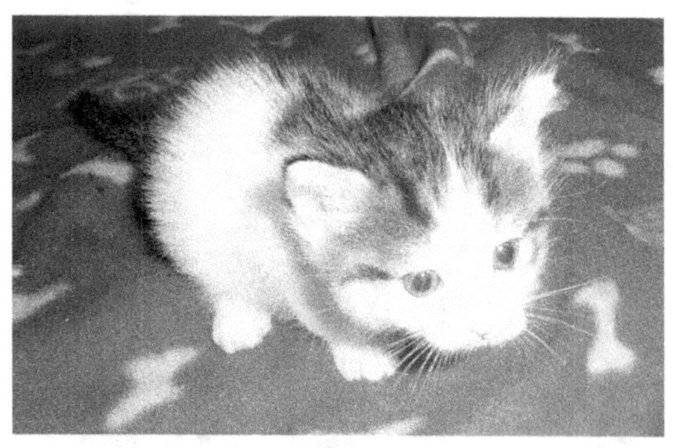

Next, little Kosmo resolved to go. He chose his mother's farmstead. He conveyed to me that he intended to make beautiful babies with the ravishing Cleopatra. Well, we will see what the folks at the stables say to that. He runs riot in and around the farm with his new friends. He has already discovered mice from the old toms. A very fine cat life. And yes: he has indeed fathered gorgeous babies. Having fulfilled his ambitions there he sought out a new abode in the village.

Timi, our little Speedy, decided for Holland. Here, his nickname was Speedy, because he sped through the house like a crazy thing.

He endured an eight-hour car journey without complaint. He slept the whole time on the car floor.

He was our little problem child and we ought to have held onto him. He did not want to do his business in the cat toilet like his sisters did. When I told him that he could not behave like this in his new home it worked.

One or two days before departure he used the cat toilet as if it were a matter of course. He is indeed a clever little chap.

He gets on very well with the lady cat of the house. He is still a wild child, a most lovable tomcat.

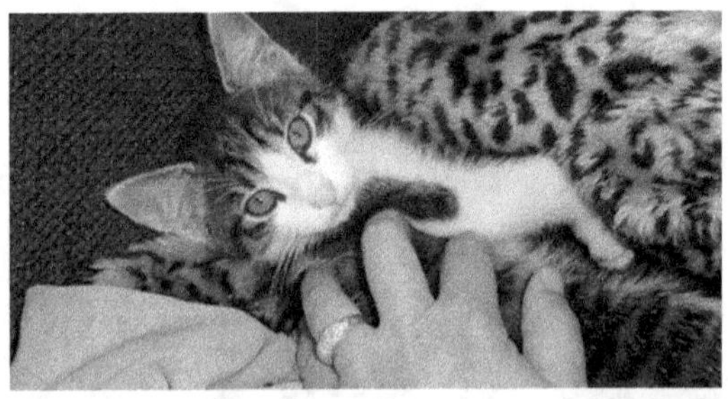

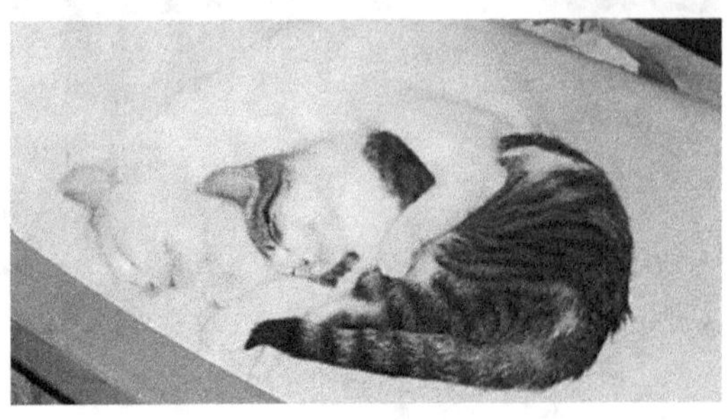

Sheela stayed with her mama and us. My beloved tom Schnaxl is embodied in her. She is all sunshine.

Little Sheela assists me with my work.

She is my transmitter, my amplifier, when I am unable to readily converse with frightened, insecure animals. She assists, boosting the signals. How this functions, I have no idea - it is a wonderful thing though, and loads of fun.

Now to the heading of this section: What do animals seek to show humans?

An example in answer to this question:
A customer's dog was insecure and afraid of being alone. Talking with the woman it emerged that she suffered that very

problem as well as suffering poor self-esteem. She caused the dog to be alive to her "problem" through her own conduct.

Often it is the interview with the animal's owner that suggests a solution.
In writing this I am made aware that my Sunshine reflects my own earlier behavior. When attacked she withdraws leaving the field to the others. This is interesting to observe.
Try it for yourself some time!

Another aspect is our fears. We hear about cancer everywhere. I have already told of the female dog diagnosed with breast cancer. The owner's partner died of the same illness. Why would it be different with this dog?

Her greatest fear was that the dog would be stricken by the illness. This "wish" was fulfilled in the form of this diagnosis. The dog showed her that it must by no means end this way. It demonstrated that there are many other possibilities.

Cats are very intelligent animals. As I have written in the section about electronic smog, cats seek radiation and dogs avoid electromagnetic radiation.

If a water vein or another source of radiation runs under your bed the cat will always go there to sleep.

If you have a dog, then observe where he likes to lie down: you will certainly sleep well there, as there are no emissions.

This can also be observed in nature.

A stork will not build its nest on a roof where there is strong radiation.

Animals flee fire; when volcanic eruption threatens they are alert. Dolphins in particular, and fish, sense geologic changes like seaquakes and tidal waves.

What does "civilized" humanity do? It concerns itself with work and the accumulation of material things. What must come to pass to change this?

It would be a positive first step if each of us begins with their pet no matter what it may be or size. Observation of our two and four-legged friends, and perhaps communication with them, would allow our coexistence to be more harmonious.

To admit something new? To move in the right direction? To discover something in respect to oneself? We make the decisions for ourselves. I wish all that possess the courage joy in discovery! Animals are such wonderful creatures: They accord humans their trust although or even though humans often treat them poorly and take advantage of this trust.

Try speaking to animals for yourself! It makes no difference whether with your own, those of friends or acquaintances, or with animals that live wild. Perhaps you will view these beings differently! Make connection via the heart and allow yourself to be surprised. Maybe these words have made you curious! I wish you great pleasure in trying this out!

14.2 How does animal communication work? A primer

As a sign of appreciation I would like to introduce you the readers of this book and particularly Daniel Peter to animal communication.

Most important in the beginning is to take the time and to stay calm. There is no advantage in attempting this in a hurry or in passing after a stressed workday. I believe that animals have earned the respect that we take sufficient time to speak to them. Likewise, it is not so effective if the television or the radio is playing in the background. Find peace both within and outwardly. Furthermore, it is crucial that your own animals do not remain in the room. This spawns a certain disquietude.

First and foremost I advise you to attempt this with animals belonging to friends, acquaintances, or neighbors. One can confirm whether the utterances are accurate. Should you not know the animal personally, it is possible to make connection by means of a photograph.

Tip: When you speak with your friend's animals do not judge the answers, or try to explain them. Pass them on to the owner just as you received them.

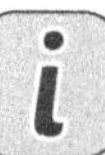

Animal communication works this way:

First sit or lie comfortably (whatever you find more agreeable). Close the eyes and breathe deeply. Breathe deep into the stomach and further down. Should many thoughts buzz round the head ask yourself: "Where will my next thought come from? Will the next thought come from the right or the left?" Mostly you will notice that the thought is gone. By this means something wonderful ensues: total calm.

The next step is to in the mind's eye visualize the animal with which you wish to speak. Contact is then made between your heart and that of the animal. This

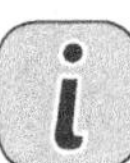

Continuation: Animal communication works this way:

connection might be looked upon as a garden hose or a tunnel of light. I often tell my course attendees that they could view the connection as being like an Internet connection: one does not see it but words travel back and forth. Do what works for you; try new ways. The heart to heart is of essence. This is also true when making connection via a photograph for the responses you receive are related to the time the photo was taken and are no longer actual. The aim is to make connection with the animal's heart.

My first question is always: "Do you … (name of the animal if known) wish to speak to me?" As I have already said: These questions and answers occur in thought only. Now it gets exciting! Is that a yes or is it no? In this context it is important to know that the first word that is sensed, comes to mind, or yes, crops up as a word, is correct! In that instant where you begin to deliberate the head kicks in. So: The initial thought is on target!

Now you can pose other questions. If the reply does not satisfy, inquire further, prod, express doubt, and where necessary reshape the question. At times people are disappointed, because they think or expect that the animal will converse as you or I might - not so. Sometimes I hear the animal speaking loud and clear, mostly though it is images, thoughts, feelings, and smells that I receive. So, be inquisitive as to the what and the how you receive!

Finally, express your appreciation, and take leave. This is how the connection is ended.

I would like to ask one more thing of you: Do this pleasurably, have fun. It is a wonderful experience that can enrich life. Best, do this without expectations or pressure - that can only inhibit communication.

14.3 How did I begin with animal communication?

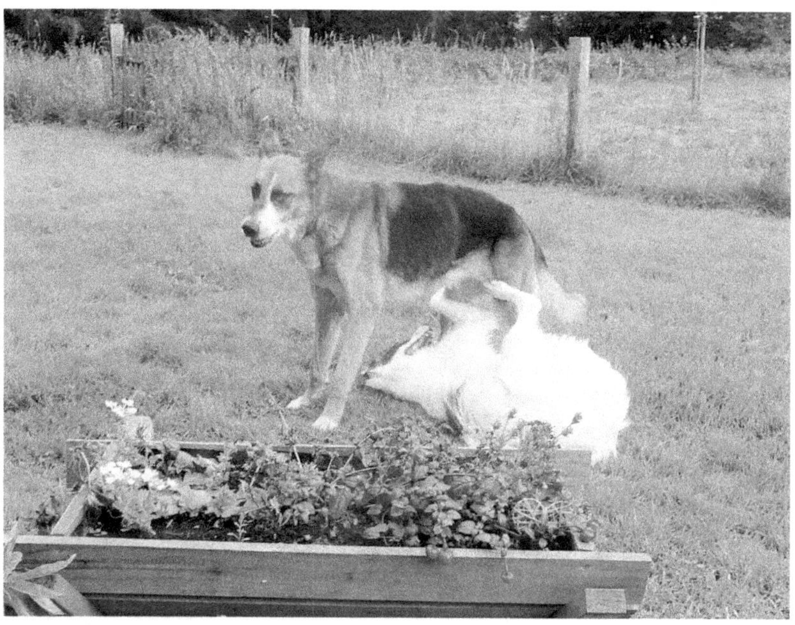

I assembled and wrote my first small booklet describing my experiences regarding "animal communication" several years ago. It is titled "How Animals See the World Through Their Eyes" (Wie die Tiere die Welt mit ihren Augen sehen), and is available from Engelsdorfer Verlag.

Bibliography

Becvar, Dr. Wolfgang. Naturheilkunde für Hunde: Grundlagen, Methoden, Krankheitsbilder, (Natural Healing for Dogs: Basics, Methods, Symptoms). Stuttgart, 2003.

Becvar, Dr. Wolfgang. Naturheilkunde für Katzen: Grundlagen, Methoden, Krankheitsbilder, (Natural Healing for Cats: Basics, Methods, Symptoms). Stuttgart, 2003.

Daubenmerkl, Wolfgang. Tierkrankheiten und ihre Behandlung: Hund, Katze, Pferd, Schwein, Rind (Animal Disorders and Their Treatment: Dogs, Cats, Horses, Swine, Cattle) Stuttgart, 2011.

Fischer, Hartmut P. A. The DMSO Handbook: A New Paradigm in Healthcare, Schnaittach 2015 (Das DMSO-Handbuch: Verborgenes Heilwissen aus der Natur). Schnaittach, 2014.

Franz, Robert. OPC - Das Fundament Menschlicher Gesundheit (OPC - The Foundation of Human Health). Rottendorf, 2014.

Grimm, Hans-Ulrich. Katzen würden Mäuse kaufen: Schwarzbuch Tierfutter (Cats Would Buy Mice: Animal Feed Black Book). Munich, 2009.

Humble, Jim. MMS: Breakthrough - The Miracle Mineral Solution of the 21st Century (2006) https://jimhumble.co, 2006

Humble, Jim. MMS: Der Durchbruch. Immenstadt, 2012.

Kalcker, Dr. Andreas. CDS/MMS: Health is Possible (CDS/MMS: Heilung ist möglich). Jim Humble Verlag: 2014.

Oswald, Dr. Antje. Das MMS-Handbuch: Gesundheit in eigener Verantwortung (The MMS Handbook: Your Health in your Hands). Schnaittach, 2011.

Wolf-Dieter Storl. Healing Lyme Disease Naturally (Borreliose natürlich heilen). Berkely, CA, 2010.

Maria Treben. Health through God's Pharmacy - Advice and Proven Cures with Medicinal Herbs, (Heilkräuter aus dem Garten Gottes: Guter Rat aus meiner Kräuterbibel für Gesundheit und Wohlbefinden). Steyr, 2013.

Yoda, Peter. Ein medizinischer Insider packt aus: Ein Dokumentarroman, (A Medical Insider Tells All: A Documentary Novel). Kernen, 2007.

Translator's note:
The titles known to be available in English translation at the time of publication are listed first; the original German language titles follow in brackets. The books that are not yet available in English appear in German first with a presumptive English title (books at times are given new titles when translated) in brackets.

16

Explanations of Abbreviations and Formulas

ppm - parts per million (3000 ppm = 0.3%)

$NaClO_2$ - Sodium chlorite

NaCl - Sodium chloride

C_2H_6OS - DMSO - Dimethyl sulfoxide

CDI - Chlorine dioxide injection

CDS/CDL - gaseous ClO_2 dissolved in water
(CDS = Chlorine dioxide solution; CDL = Chlordioxidlösung in German)

CDSplus - preserved CDS

OPC - Oligomeric procyanidin

ClO_2 - Chlorine dioxide

HCl - Hydrochloric acid

$C_4H_6O_6$ - Tartaric acid

$C_6H_8O_7$ - Citric acid

$C_3H_6O_3$ - Lactic acid

17
Acknowledgements

I would like to thank some dear people who have assisted me along the way. It took a long time to write this book. Hence there are matters that slipped into the background at home, or were left unattended. For this reason I would like to give thanks to my wonderful husband Rene. At times he did not get the attention he deserved. As with this book, he has backed me up from the inception with all of my projects. He has always been a great support. He was the first to read the individual chapters of this book, and I am forever thankful for his honest opinions.

Another very dear person I wish to acknowledge here is Daniel Peter, who trusted in me, brought this project to being, and offered substantial encouragement.

Naturally, I must thank the lovely Gabriela who first brought me in contact with the publisher. You are simply wonderful people!

And I owe a very special thank you to the animals that as patients so trustingly put themselves in my/our hands. Of course I am grateful to our own animals, who at times did not receive sufficient attention, or whose walks were cut short.

I wish to convey loving gratitude to my friend Helga. Together with her I went through turbulent times as an employee representative, and was able to learn much of advantage to me.

Even today I must smile at her many long sentences incorporating many, many commas. I hope that her dream of writing a book be realized soon, that she finds the time necessary.

Another special thanks you to Petra. She taught me "how to walk" in the domain of animal communication, and provided the requisite reassurance when I was in need. Thank you for being there!

Three more marvelous, creative people deserve thanks: The editor and author Monika Stolina-Wolf, layout artist and graphic designer Eva Saarbourg, and graphic artist Markus Hoffmann. Thank you that you did not lose patience, and for producing this fantastic piece!

I am grateful for this project and the experience garnered as a result. While working on this book I read and researched a great deal sparking genuine advances in my development, and much more.

Thanks to you dear readers for being interested in and responsive to this book, and that you have acquired it. My hope is that the reading it has brought you pleasure and that the content is of assistance.

Monika Rekelhof
February 2015

18
List of Practitioners

To follow are some therapeutic practices for animals and therapists with experience of MMS and who readily assist animal owners treat their animals autonomously. They will willingly shed light on MMS and explain the possibilities and risks.

Legal Information: It is neither possible nor permissible to guarantee recovery. MMS is authorized for the disinfection of water only. It cannot be prescribed or required. MMS is not an officially recognized "medicine." Nobody can prevent you from administering MMS yourself though; just as making compresses with the similarly officially unauthorized "medicine" vinegar cannot be prohibited.

Needless to say, you may make contact with these people in order to arrange an appointment.

If you yourself are a veterinarian, an alternative practitioner for animals, or therapist, and wish to appear in this listing in forthcoming editions please contact the publisher.

Germany

Heilpraktikerin für Mensch und Tier / Alternative Practitioner for Humans and Animals
Sylke Georgoulis
Baden Württemberg
Heilpraxis für klassische Homöopathie und Naturheilkunde / Baden Württemberg Naturopathic Practice for Homeopathy and Natural Medicine
sg@heilpraxiskarlsruhe.de
mobile: 01 77 / 421 55 48

Tierheilerin und Tierkommunikatorin / Animal Healer and Animal Communicator
Susanne Robers-Gerigk
Alternative Heilmittel für Mensch und Tier / Alternative Medicine for Humans and Animals
46325 Borken
s-r-g@web.de
mobile: 01 76 / 32 07 10 17

Heilerin / Healer
Claudia Bornschein
Spyckweg 3
46495 Rees
www.REIKI-NRW.net
Info@reiki-nrw.net
mobile: 01 74 / 659 63 64

Tierheilpraxis Angel-Ranch / Angel Ranch Therapeutic Practice for Horses and Dogs
Michaela von Jähnichen
Seulbitzerstr. 7
95466 Weidenberg/Neunkirchen
mobile: 01 70 / 2 86 16 56
mail@angel-ranch.de

Mobile Tierheilpraxis Schiller für Groß- und Kleintiere / Mobile Therapeutic Practice for Humans and Animals
Stefanie Schiller
Archfeldstr. 16
99831 Ifta
mobile: 01 62 / 945 32 28

Gesundheitspraxis für Mensch und Tier / Health Practice for Humans and Animals
Karin Rutka
Ingoldinger Str. 3
88427 Bad Schussenried
Tel.: 07583-2227
karin.rutka@freenet.de
www.karin-rutka.de

Austria / Österreich

Therapeutin / Therapist
Eva Hautz
Bradl 321
A – 6210 Wiesing
Tel.: 00 43 / 650-303 31 13
E-Mail: info@healing-horses.at
www.healing-horses.at

19
Blue Socks

*T*his book was actually complete and I had begun with the first corrections when I read the ensuing story. It would not leave me be. It saddened me and gave me pause, just how we are manipulated and how very often we ourselves facilitate this.

The same happens as regards our animals. When I see advertising for chew-bone to counter tartar, feed for this problem, supplements for that, I can only shake my head. When do the red horse blankets to prevent laminitis, yellow dog collars to cure hip dysplasia, or the cuddly, blue, anti cat flu blankets appear on the market?

Maybe you are laughing and thinking: "The very idea!" But is this so improbable?

Here then is the story from the book "A Medical Insider Tells All" (Ein medizinischer Insider packt aus) by Peter Yoda.

"Blue Socks Against Cancer

Picture this: Your intention is to establish a market for 'health socks.' You must begin by commissioning a study. All men with let's say prostate gland cancer are asked the color of their socks. Whatever you decide to research, one group will certainly fare better than the other. Assume that 6% of those in the group who wear blue socks survive, and those in the group wearing red only 3%. For your advertising (printed of course on glossy paper, and the study is needless to say presented to the medical professionals at a five-star hotel) the result is: Blue socks give rise to an improved survival rate of 50%! Now all that is required is an academic (known in our circles as a 'Mouth for Hire' = Mietmaul) to explain WHY the blue socks live longer. One could then say that blue socks radiate at a wavelength range between 490 - 450 nm, and that the latest research from the USA (always sounds impressive) confirms that in laboratory tests prostate cancer cells that have been exposed to such emissions are destroyed more rapidly. Do not forget to append the all-important statement: This research must of course be augmented, though first indications are so encouraging that we hope to be able to introduce the optimal "anti-cancer socks" to the market in the foreseeable future.

What is so absurd is that with this kind of study there is no need to falsify the research, the data, or the findings: All that is promulgated is almost true!

The like has been foisted on cancer patients for years. One needs only replace the term 'socks' with chemotherapy, radiotherapy, calcium antagonist, Beta blocker, GM technology, et cetera, et cetera.

You understand the rationale!"

*It requires great skill to administer
a substance to treat an illness,
but the supreme skill is to know
when to forgo such treatment.*

Philippe Pinel

20
Keyword Index

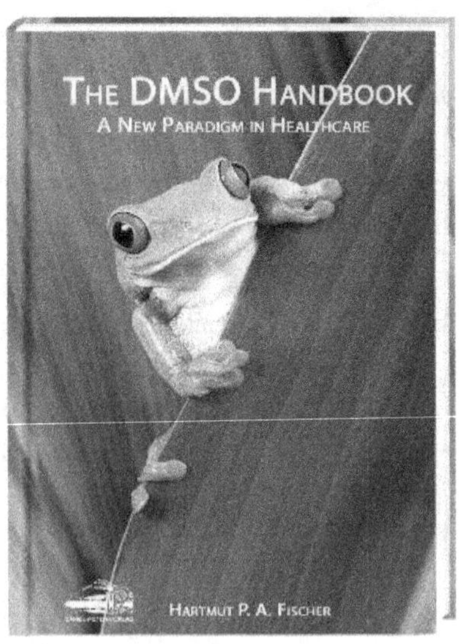

The DMSO Handbook

by

Dr. rer. nat. Hartmut Fischer

DMSO, an easily accessible universal therapeutic agent, is currently enjoying a remarkable comeback in the field of alternative medicine after having been treasured for many years by just a small number of insiders. It has mainly become known as a fast-acting, well-tolerated treatment for acute inflammations and traumatic injuries. It has an anti-inflammatory effect, it relieves pain immediately, it accelerates the swift resorption of swellings and haemorrhages, and it supports wound healing. But DMSO does much more. This natural substance is an extremely useful basis for therapeutic self-reliance and a huge leap towards freedom from the many side effects caused by standard medications.

Dr Hartmut Fischer is a scientist and alternative health practitioner. In this book, he draws upon many years of experience of working with DMSO, both in a scientific capacity as well as in his role as a health professional.

292 pages. Hardback. ISBN 978-3-9815255-1-9

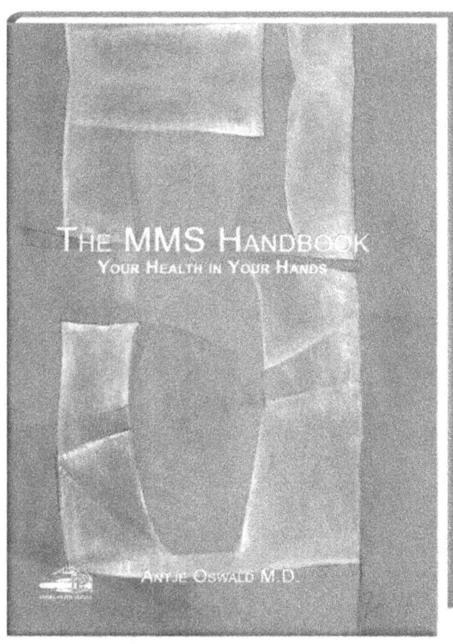

The comprehensive new reference book on MMS

Will MMS revolutionise the way many diseases are treated?

MMS – an amazing substance that consists of three atoms – can eliminate a large number of pathogens. Until now users could only draw from the experiences of a small number of brave pioneers. In this book a medical doctor addresses the subject of MMS for the first time. Dr Antje Oswald, a general practitioner in Detmold, Germany, has been intensively engaged in researching the effects of MMS and presents the fruits of that work here.

Take advantage of her knowledge and insights and discover the numerous possibilities of this phenomenal substance!

"Very readable and with plenty of depth to satisfy my thirst for details. Most importantly, it includes clear, detailed instructions for self-responsible readers on how to make use of MMS. This book has all the ingredients necessary to guarantee it a permanent place in the field of alternative medicine."
Uwe Karstädt, Alternative practitioner and author

"Thank you for the new MMS book! It has turned out fantastically and is an exciting read. Congratulations! May many people profit from it. I am delighted to recommend it to others. Great book!"
Dr Sophia Papadopoulou, General Practitioner

Paperback, 275 pages, ISBN 978-3-9815255-3-3

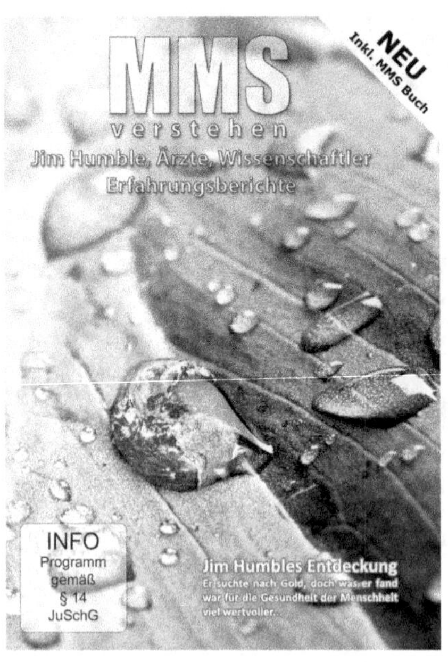

The documentary film
MMS verstehen / Understanding MMS
on DVD
fourth revised edition!

Audio in English / German / Spanish

This film imparts a deeper understanding of MMS. It features doctors, scientists and users, and you will meet in it some of the people mentioned in The MMS Handbook, such as Jim Humble, Dr John Humiston and Clara Beltrones.
The efficacy of MMS is documented using numerous first-hand reports. It is truly inspiring to learn how people have used MMS to cure serious and refractory illnesses.

Now in a fourth revised edition with:

– a 16-page booklet (in German only) which includes interesting articles on MMS, and detailed usage instructions for the most common MMS sets on the market today

– a bonus video on structured water and the surprising effect of structured water on plants.

Format DVD9. Playing time: 105 minutes. Languages: English, German, Spanish.   ISBN 978-3-9812917-0-4. Price Euros 28.00

For more information visit www.daniel-peter-verlag.de

www.ingramcontent.com/pod-product-compliance
Lightning Source LLC
LaVergne TN
LVHW060554200726
843509LV00003B/117